I Know You Like to Smoke

But You Can Quit—Now

THE EXPERIMENT

BECAUSE EVERY BOOK IS A TEST OF NEW IDEAS

I Know
You Like
to Smoke

But You
Can Quit—
Now

Andreas Jopp

THE EXPERIMENT
NEW YORK

I Know You Like To Smoke, But You Can Quit—Now
Copyright © Andreas Jopp, 2014
Translation by Colin McCullough, Thessaloniki, Greece
Graphics courtesy Peter Palm, Berlin, Germany
Cartoons on pages 130, 132, 133 courtesy Marek Blaha, Offenbach, Germany
Photograph on page 88 © Sergey Ash/shutterstock.com
Photograph on page 187 © sergign/shutterstock.com

The Experiment, LLC
220 East 23rd Street • Suite 301
New York, NY 10010-4674
www.theexperimentpublishing.com

The Experiment's books are available at special discounts when purchased in bulk for premiums and sales promotions as well as for fundraising or educational use. For details, contact us at info@theexperimentpublishing.com.

Many of the designations used by manufacturers and sellers to distinguish their products are claimed as trademarks. Where those designations appear in this book and The Experiment was aware of a trademark claim, the designations have been capitalized.

Library of Congress Cataloging-in-Publication Data

Jopp, Andreas.
 I know you like to smoke, but you can quit : now / Andreas Jopp.
    pages cm
 Includes bibliographical references.
 ISBN 978-1-61519-089-8 (pbk.) -- ISBN 978-1-61519-180-2 (ebook)
 1. Smoking--Psychological aspects. 2. Smoking cessation. I. Title.
 BF789.S6J67 2014
 616.86'506--dc23

                              2013047110

ISBN 978-1-61519-089-8
ebook ISBN 978-1-61519-180-2

Cover design by Howard Grossman
Front cover photograph © hriana/Fotolia
Interior Cover photographs, ©Vladyslav Danilin/shutterstock.com, © Elnur/shutterstock.com, © Jason Stitt/shutterstock.com, © nrt/shutterstock.com, ©arahan/Fotolia, © GlobalStock/iStockphoto.com
Text design by Pauline Neuwirth, Neuwirth & Associates, Inc.

Manufactured in the United States of America
Distributed by Workman Publishing Company, Inc.
Distributed simultaneously in Canada by Thomas Allen and Son Ltd.
First printing March 2014
10 9 8 7 6 5 4 3 2 1

Disclaimer

This publication intends to provide helpful and informative material on the subjects addressed in the publication. It is sold in the understanding that the author and publisher are not engaged in rendering medical, health, psychological, psychiatric, or any other kind of personal professional services in the book. The reader should consult his or her medical, health, or other competent professional before adopting any of the suggestions in this book or drawing references from it. When *you* quit the drug nicotine, you need to consult an experienced doctor or psychiatrist, especially if you suffer from mood swings, self-aggression or aggressions against others, or any other physical or unusual mental condition. The author and the publisher disclaim all responsibility for all liabilities, loss, or risk, personal or otherwise, which is incurred as a consequence, directly or indirectly, of the use and application of any of the concerns of this book.

Only you and an experienced doctor of your choice can decide whether you want to take medication or nicotine replacement products. Medical advice can only be given by a doctor who has a chance to personally observe and understand your health condition and objectives. The information given in this book is solely intended for information purposes and should not be taken for medical advice. While the information has been researched with best knowledge, science does uncover new insights and thereby the information of this book may become obsolete quickly. Neither the author nor the publisher assumes any legal liability or responsibility for the completeness, the usefulness, or the future accuracy of the information. By virtue of this Disclaimer and Warning you may not hold us responsible for any adverse or side effect you suffer and you may not look to us to indemnify you from your own free decision to use or not use nicotine replacement products or medications that have to be prescribed and monitored by a doctor.

Contents

Introduction   ix

How Do the Book Plus Internet Program
Work Together?   xxiv

PART 1: DO YOU "LIKE" TO SMOKE?   1

1 From "Liking" to "Having" to Smoke   3
2 Advertisements and Hollywood as Role Models   20
3 How Nicotine Dealers Get You Hooked   29
4 The Biochemistry of Happiness   37
5 My Dog, My Children, My Wife . . . :
   The Uncomfortable Pressure of the Passive Smoker   45

PART 2: SMOKING AND THE MIND   53

6 The Daily Ups and Downs Caused by Nicotine   55
7 Smoking with No Advantages: Relaxation, Stress
   Reduction, and Improvement of Mood   69
8 The Stimulation and Concentration Myth   86
9 Stress and Mood: When You Started,
   When You're Quitting   97
10 Interview with Prof. Parrott—Smoking and the Mind   113
11 The Power of Conditioning   126
12 Your Cigarette Brand and Other Smokers   143

PART 3: OTHER REASONS TO QUIT SMOKING   147

13 Weight and Beauty   149
14 The Daily Cocktail of Chemicals   154

15 The Dewy-Eyed View of Risks 167
16 Things Do Get Better! 175
17 What Are You Going to Decide? 178

PART 4: BECOME A NONSMOKER AND
         MAINTAIN YOUR WEIGHT 189

18 Smoking Doesn't Keep You Slim 191
19 Addiction and the Sweet Tooth 201
20 How to Avoid the Roly-Poly Trap 206
21 Protein—Feeling Full and Happy 219
22 Maintain Your Weight After You Quit Smoking:
    The Shopping List 225

PART 5: THE MOST SUCCESSFUL STRATEGIES
         FOR QUITTING 233

23 How to Become Smoke-*Free* 235
24 Hypnotherapy—Communicating with
    Your Unconscious 239
25 Nicotine Replacement Therapy—
    An Aid or a Business? 253
26 Acupuncture—Faith Doesn't Move Mountains 267
27 Chantix—Reconquering the Receptors That Make
    You Happy 269
28 The Last Cigarette 276
29 Strategies to Avoid Slips and Lapses 279
30 Your Personal Care and Support 291

Login and Password for the Online Program 294
A Final Word 295
Endnotes 297
About the Author 307

Introduction

HOW OFTEN HAVE YOU SAID TO yourself, "I like smoking" and "I can quit whenever I want." Like most smokers, I've often used both statements in various forms. Whenever someone thought he had to draw me into a sort of smoker's interrogation, with an all-inclusive, subsequent debate, I used to cut him short with these 2 sentences and be at peace. But, of course, all smokers know that these 2 statements are both true and false at the same time.

If it weren't true that 1 out of 4 smokers dies from the consequences of "liking" to smoke, then we would never think about quitting—because with a cigarette, for a brief moment, you just feel good. You're more relaxed, less stressed, and calmer. For a moment, you can just unwind. Unfortunately, after 45 minutes, the nicotine level drops so much that you feel like having another. The fact that I was ruining my health repeatedly brought me into the typical "smoker's conflict": I would quickly skim over information about the supposed damage to one's health, refute it internally with a few spurious arguments, and then repress it so I could keep on smoking. Think about it—have you ever offered your children a cigarette? Probably not. Even the most passionate smoker wouldn't do that. So, maybe we don't enjoy smoking so wholeheartedly after all. How would you react if your daughter began to smoke? Would you say, "That's wonderful. I've always liked smoking myself"? That doesn't seem to sound right, either. So it becomes clear just how ambivalent "liking" to smoke really is. Most smokers would prefer to quit, if only they knew a simple and reliable method.

The second statement, "I can quit whenever I want," is true, too. Of course, you *could* quit whenever you wanted. But after my own umpteen spontaneous attempts, it was clear to me that this must be something that applied to smokers with stronger willpower. And I had absolutely no desire to spill the beans about this to a nonsmoker, who would draw me once again into a long interrogation from which I would emerge frustrated and with lower self-esteem. Even though I didn't manage to quit, I invented this excuse for myself: "I smoke of my own volition and apparently I just don't really want to quit yet. Of course, I can quit at any time . . ."

And so, for 20 years, I guiltily "liked" to smoke and "could have quit" if only I'd "really wanted to." But all during those 20 years, *now* was just never the right time.

How Many Cigarettes Do You Smoke?

Adding up the cigarettes I was actually smoking, I tended to round the numbers down. I had everything under control. Like all smokers, "I didn't smoke a lot"—"just 5 to 10 cigarettes a day"—if anyone asked me. That never harmed anyone. I "never smoked at home" . . . except when I watched television (frequently) or was on the phone (even more frequently). Anyway, "I never smoked when I was working on the computer" . . . except when I was stressed out (daily) or had to write a difficult text and concentrate (pretty often, as an author). When something got on my nerves (now and again) or my mood wasn't the best (happens to us all), then I really enjoyed a cigarette. When I was waiting for a train or sitting in a traffic jam, I often . . . well . . . (as an exception) had a cigarette. Having a cigarette while waiting gave me something to do (though we all know trains are usually punctual . . . and traffic jams are virtually unknown). Sometimes I smoked a few more, such as when I was going out (but that was only 2 or 3 times a week). That would add maybe 5 or 6 cigarettes to the tally. And, maybe a pack on the weekends, occasionally. But, of course, only to be social. And I was smoking, above all, for enjoyment. By that I mean I *always* had one with a cup of coffee, after eating, with a beer, in the pub, after sex, to relax, to perk up, after breakfast, during breaks . . . but just to enjoy. Actually, I should have been completely happy, having had so much enjoyment. Okay, there were a few—and I mean just a few— cigarettes that I smoked on autopilot, without thinking. When others lit up, or for no particular reason at all. I guess if you were to add it all up, it couldn't have been more than 5 or 10 of those. Let's say 15, at the most. On rare occasions, perhaps 20 to 25. But only now and again, of course. All right, so it was more often than that. But I was never addicted! I had smoked for the pleasure of it since I was 16. I smoked because I enjoyed it, and liked it—most of the time.

I think a lot of smokers go through the same thing. In the evening, you're appalled when the pack is empty. "Damn, only one left," so you step out quickly: "Better get another pack . . . just to be on the safe side. But I'm not addicted; I *like* smoking."

Do You Always Like Smoking?

Probably not, otherwise you wouldn't have bought this book. Maybe you already have 3 or 4 failed attempts to quit under your belt. You may hate smoking, now and again, and as time passes, ever more frequently: When you "have to" smoke and there are no cigarettes in the house. When you find yourself driving to the nearest gas station at the most impossible times to go get them. When you wake up in the morning with a throbbing headache, the typical smoker's hangover, after a smoke-filled night of partying. When you cough up sticky phlegm in the morning. When you stand outside the office or your own home, smoking in the cold once again. When there is an irritating nonsmoker beside you. When you have the feeling you need a cigarette *now* but you can't and—worse yet—can't get your mind off it. When you don't have the courage to quit and this eats away at your self-confidence. It's then that you find that you actually hate smoking. As time passed, I, like all other smokers, just started "liking to smoke" less and less. The only thing I couldn't fathom was how to get a grip on my "needing to smoke." Naturally, you keep such doubts to yourself. The mental to-and-fro is your own affair and nobody else's business.

In fact, you would prefer not to smoke if you didn't have that vague feeling that it would be unbelievably frustrating to not smoke in certain situations. And life would surely become less enjoyable. Certainly you would miss smoking. And, in any case, it would be really difficult to quit forever. Most smokers are forever torn between the wish to quit and the wish to enjoy. So they just continue to smoke until such times as when perhaps some revelation dawns on them that the time to quit has come. That is the hope. Most smokers will wait decades for such a revelation. Perhaps 10 years later, $30,000 poorer, and with a chronic smoker's cough, you might be ready.

Only few smokers are so indecisive in other areas of their lives. Most smokers know exactly what they don't want, at the very least, and also see things through that are important to them, in both their professional and private lives. But smoking is a different matter: Why do so many smokers want to quit and yet continue to smoke? What is it that makes smoking so enjoyable? Why do we lose control over smoking? Why are we so afraid to quit?

How can *you* break away from cigarettes in the best way, *if* you decide to make that break? I say intentionally "*if* you decide" because I assume you want to first browse through this book, and that you're still not positive whether you really want to quit. At least, that's what I've kept in mind while writing this book. Be critical. Don't believe anything I've written until I've proven it to you. As a start, I think it's great you've decided to have a closer look at quitting. Congratulations.

Most Smokers Quit Sooner or Later

Let's step outside the United States for a moment: In Germany, there are exactly as many ex-smokers as there are smokers—30% are ex-smokers and 30% are smokers. All of these ex-smokers have managed to get off nicotine! "Well, okay," you may say, "1 in 2 managed to quit. So my chances are 50–50." Wrong. Many more were able to quit! We need to factor in that tobacco companies are continuously recruiting children and youth, increasing the total number of smokers. But over time most smokers stop. In the 1970s (the generation that is now in its 60s), 60% of German men smoked. Of this generation, however, only 13% continue to smoke. Many more than half managed to quit! In fact, 79% of smokers manage to quit during their lifetime—nearly 8 out of 10 smokers. This shows very different statistics—and you could be one of them!

In the United States, Australia, or Great Britain, even more smokers are successful at quitting. In the United States, only 19% of the population smokes; in California, only 12%. Aggressive antismoking legislation and tobacco taxes have made smoking unattractive, and support programs help smokers when they are ready to quit. The important message is: Quit now. Anybody can make it.

Are Ex-smokers Unhappier?

You may say, "Those ex-smokers are missing out on something, for sure . . . I never want to go without a cigarette after a meal." But such smokers haven't only managed to quit—they don't even feel as if they are missing out on something. Otherwise, with nearly a third of the German population being ex-smokers, you would expect to constantly hear how much they miss the pleasure of a cigarette and what a permanent loss not smoking is. But this is not the case. Take my experience from talking to ex-smokers who have been off of cigarettes for a year or two: 99% waste so little thought on cigarettes that they don't even find the need to mention that they had ever smoked.

Major surveys of ex-smokers show that they rate their lives as happy or even happier, but by no means do they rate it as less happy or less satisfying.[1] But you don't have to take my word for this. Unlike other authors, I won't try to talk you into believing that you will be happier without cigarettes only because that happened to be the case with me. I will continually show you studies of thousands of smokers and ex-smokers to rid you of the uncertainty and fear of quitting. You can learn so much from ex-smokers! How did these smokers feel when they quit? What preconceptions did they have about quitting?

"Are my fears justified that I might always feel I am missing something?" You should know this precisely before you decide to quit. And like most smokers after a short period, you very likely will discover that you do not regret quitting and that you won´t miss anything. You can read more about this in chapter 9.

Nicotine—Your Physical Dependence

Of course, you are convinced that this is going to be completely different for you and that it will be awfully difficult to get unhooked from nicotine. Nearly every smoker who wants to quit feels like this. However, "It wasn't easy but much easier than I imagined" is a very typical experience of many smokers who quit. Uncertainty and fear stop us from risking the first step. With regard to most of these concerns, the expectations and fears of smokers are very similar. This is due to the way nicotine affects the brain. As soon as nicotine is broken down and leaves the brain, it creates a diffuse feeling of restlessness. In extreme cases, it can even cause fear and panic when the nicotine level in the bloodstream falls substantially. Your brain's biochemistry recovers quickly after quitting and panic and fear subside completely.

Many people smoke to relieve stress, to concentrate, to relax, or to enhance their mood. But do cigarettes really help reduce stress? Does smoking make you more focused or more stimulated; does it improve your mood? If so, then smoking would have its benefits, and logically, quitting would then mean missing out on these. Smokers are totally convinced of this. Of course you smoke because of these benefits—why else? The bottom line is that your brain's dependence on nicotine *causes* more stress, restlessness, and changes in mood and energy levels. That means that smoking has no benefit. A few weeks after quitting, once your brain has recovered from its addiction, you will feel more resistant to stress, more relaxed, and overall in better form. Reputable scientists have looked into precisely this issue in many studies of smokers and ex-smokers. And the results are really amazing! Read more about this in chapter 8.

Conditioning—Your Psychological Dependence

Nicotine causes not only physical dependence by modifying the biochemistry of the brain, but under the influence of nicotine, we closely connect in our mind certain situations with smoking.

These triggers—known in psychology as conditioning—make us automatically grab a cigarette; for example, while having a cup of coffee, when others are smoking, with alcohol, after eating . . . And then we reach for a cigarette, "just like that," for no apparent reason at all. These conditioned responses are totally independent of the nicotine level in our body. Take a close, conscious look at other smokers. You will be amazed at how automatic and unconscious these smoking triggers are, which cause a smoker to light up. Conditioned triggers are much more than a habit. They are a fixed behavior and it takes time to get rid of them.

Emotional situations can have exactly the same effect in triggering the desire for a cigarette. If you are stressed or in a bad mood—you know exactly how a cigarette can rid you of this feeling. And taking 70,000 puffs a year enforces this conditioning again and again. Many smokers have asked themselves, even across a lifetime, why they feel like another cigarette immediately after they have just put one out. It is only recently that we have discovered how this conditioning works in triggering the desire to smoke. This is the main reason that we continue to smoke and why nicotine makes us so dependent. Chapter 11 is a real eye-opener on this topic.

Having the Patience to Relearn

When you are physically clean of nicotine—and this occurs only a few days after quitting—the smoking cues that you have learned must be unlearned one by one, or deconditioned. Now for the good news: Once you've overcome this brainwashing, you will also lose the urge to smoke: A good meal will not be enhanced with a cigarette afterward and the coffee is just as stimulating without smoking. You won't waste a thought on desiring cigarettes. Millions of ex-smokers can testify to this— just as, before you started smoking, you never thought for a second to improve the taste of ice cream or a piece of cake or a side of French fries by inhaling smoke!

The Conjuring Tricks of Nicotine

A prerequisite for quitting is to understand the conjuring tricks of nicotine. It is nicotine that makes you believe that cigarettes taste good or make you feel better. These sensations are completely real. However, in actuality, you are smoking to counter the restlessness and emptiness of the nicotine withdrawal symptoms. You smoke to feel better . . . from the low state that nicotine, itself, has placed you in.

You don't need to agree with this now! But once you have figured out the mechanism, then it will be that much easier to decide to get out of this vicious cycle—to no longer let nicotine control you. Just read the book with an open mind and be ready for new things.

Please Continue Smoking!

I'm not here to persuade you to do anything! Nor should you let yourself be put under pressure by your partner or anyone else. This is only about you! And you *may and you should* continue smoking while reading this book. It is important to me that you feel totally relaxed when reading.

Please do not reduce the number of cigarettes you smoke. That just puts you under unnecessary pressure and makes each cigarette seem more important than the previous one.

There is another reason that I would like you to continue smoking. This is the only way you can take a close look at your smoking behavior and that of other smokers, without being sidetracked by craving a cigarette. The more you know about when you smoke, what typical emotional triggers make you smoke, what you personally enjoy about smoking, what you detest about smoking, why you might think of quitting, and what your fears are about quitting, the easier quitting will become.

Use the Internet Program

The accompanying interactive online learning program, with which you can create your own smoking profile, will help you choose to quit and follow through (see page xxiv for more about the interactive program). I can pose important questions and give you a lot of food for thought, but only you alone can give the right answers. Please, make use of the learning program. Make time for this. It is nothing less than your *life* we are talking about. It could be one of the most far-reaching decisions you make. One of your most important projects. Should you then decide to smoke your last cigarette, the answers you have provided will help you enormously. Why? In the course of the first weeks after quitting, you really must remind yourself exactly what you wanted to attain—regardless of the whispers coming from your addicted brain. That is how you will succeed.

An Additional Motivation: Health

In this book, I will not be confronting you with horror stories about your health. This wouldn't help. On the contrary, it would only build up resistance. You can read for yourself on cigarette packs that smoking damages your health. And has this made you quit? No, it only gets on your nerves. Only a tiny part of this book deals with the health aspect. Maybe about 5 pages. There, I do address how smokers fall into a dewy-eyed comparison of risks and start to make up their homemade personal observations so as to continue smoking ("Well, pollution is just as dangerous as smoking" . . . "Nothing is going to happen to me" . . . "My uncle smokes and he is 85" . . . followed, of course, by the classic "You have to die of something"; the question is only when and how?). I present to you the real risks to you as a smoker. Here, we have a lot of precise figures. For any other decision you would make that would have a major impact on your future, wouldn't you first seek out relevant information? So, why not here? Of course, as a smoker, you would prefer to avoid this information so as to happily continue smoking. But suppressing your fears about your own health takes up a lot of your energy. In your unconscious, the fears remain very much alive and require constant effort to keep them at bay. And even worse, they gnaw away at your self-esteem, because you know exactly what you are doing to yourself.

Nonsmokers in particular always believe you could quit smoking by endless discussion of the reasons it would be better not to smoke. But, of course, this is not the way things work. Obviously, you don´t smoke for the reasons you shouldn´t, but for the reasons that you "like" smoking. Which means that you really have to take a closer look at the reasons you do smoke. Without getting to the roots of the "I like to smoke" issue, you will always defend the advantages of smoking, instead of quitting once and for all, without regrets. So, this book is about taking a deep look inward at your own motivations: Does smoking really enhance your quality of life? Does it truly make you feel better? Only when you've found the answers to such questions will I give you a little motivational nudge about your health. Simply because, like everyone else, you want to live longer and feel younger. Yes, your addicted brain will quietly whisper in your ear that you should "enjoy the here and now" and that "we all have to die of something." But buried deep in your unconscious mind, your survival instinct is stronger. You cannot trick your unconscious. You have always known: Living longer is more important than smoking longer! But perhaps you just haven't known how you could actually go about achieving this.

Looking at the consequences of smoking initially triggers

stress and fear. Some people even need to smoke a couple of more cigarettes to suppress the stress they feel with additional nicotine. That is perfectly okay. But then this knowledge begins to form a larger picture, and a hard look at reality can motivate you even more to quit.

Quitting Without Gaining Weight

One of the main reasons that many people are hesitant to quit smoking is the fear of putting on weight. But does smoking really keep you slim? Or do we gain weight because we previously smoked? Do the statistics show that smokers are slimmer than nonsmokers? The actual findings are amazing!

Why do you feel hungry after quitting? Why do sweets reinforce addictive behaviors and make you more prone to relapse? What is the real story behind relapse and weight gain? How do you manage not to put on weight after you quit?

Not gaining weight is easy and can be done with little extra effort. Trust me: I have been writing about nutrition for over 20 years. My books are translated into 14 languages. I do *not* intend to change your eating habits. It is simply a matter of maintaining your current weight, which will for several reasons also make it easier for you to quit. My methods to maintain weight are convenient and practical (see chapters 18 through 22). Yet in all the antismoking books I have read, not a single one of them really looks at how to avoid putting on weight after quitting.

Your Perception of Smoking

What would it take for you to take a cold, hard look at your views on yourself as a smoker and the smoking culture in general? Doing so is extremely important; otherwise, in the future you will always have a feeling of nostalgia over the time when you smoked. We are talking about the social aspects of smoking. For me personally, smoking and socializing were one and the same thing. I wanted to be part of the club. For me, it was a perfectly natural part of my culture. I always identified with other smokers: "Smokers are cooler and nicer people." Every smoker believes in his or her own "smoker's personality" and has a certain image of how he or she is seen as a smoker. However, the older you get, the more independent you become of group identity and advertising slogans, which are more fitting to youngsters that have just started to smoke. That is why most smokers quit between the ages of 40 and 50.

With the maturity you possess today, look back again at when you started to smoke. How was your perspective of smoking influenced by years of exposure to advertising, film, or television? How did the cigarette industry lure you into smoking as a child or adolescent? How were smokers lied to for decades about nicotine's not being addictive? How does the nicotine industry manipulate the addiction through additives? How did the industry rig the research findings on the health risks, through biased and subsidized research (so the nicotine dealers could claim that there are "differing, controversial expert opinions")? How has the tobacco lobby bribed politicians and scientists?

All this information, taken together, can bring you to the point where you say, "Enough is enough. I quit" or "I won't allow myself to be manipulated any longer." This awakening to how you have been lied to and manipulated is a small but important part of your decision to kick cigarettes forever. Smoking has played an important part in your life. Now, nicotine-free, you can open a new and exciting chapter in your life.

You Have Nothing to Lose; You Can Only Gain

"The slower I read, the later I have to stop." You are not forced to do anything. You alone decide if you want to continue smoking or not. Maybe at the end of the book you simply want to quit. One piece of advice: Read through this book quickly. This is the best way to condense all the information you want to have to make the decision that is right for you. Now you are just gathering information. That is a positive action. In one go, you can take a look at all the jigsaw pieces and see how they fit together. Nothing more, nothing less.

Of course, we would all prefer to leave things the way they are, for changes in life are accompanied by fears. But fear of the unknown is what is setting the limits to your life. Moreover, remind yourself that you are not giving up something, but are starting something new. That is a completely different feeling. Instead of leaving something behind, you can look forward to new things. Within a short period of time, you have a life where you can cope better with stress and become more emotionally stable. Look forward to becoming more fit and having more energy every day. Fears you may have about your health disappear and unleash new energy. Your self-esteem increases because you have managed to quit. Because you have conquered your fear. Because you have escaped the smoker's trap and reclaimed your freedom.

This could be the most important decision of your life. You have nothing to lose. In the worst-case scenario, you will continue to smoke just as you do now. The best case is that you could increase your life span by 14 years. As many as that? Yes, on average, smokers' lives are shortened by 14 years by continuing to smoke just 20 cigarettes a day until they die.

Every day, you do things that show that you plan for the future and really expect to be around for a long time to come. You put on your seat belt in the car, you sign insurance contracts, you pay your mortgage, and you look forward to having grandchildren. So, you are not in the slightest indifferent to your future. Take the chance to use this book and the website to look at things from a different perspective. With an open mind. Then you can make the decision whether you would "like" to continue smoking or to try something new. Millions of ex-smokers have quit and will confirm: You will enjoy your life at least as much or even more without nicotine. You won´t miss out on anything.

> *Nothing in life is to be feared, it is only to be understood.*
> —Marie Curie

How Do the Book Plus Internet Program Work Together?

This Is How the Book Works

Smoking is as complex a behavior as a puzzle. Otherwise, millions of people would not fall into the nicotine trap and then, after several decades and some $60,000 to $70,000 less in their pockets, plus ruined health, manage to escape. I will demystify and take apart the smoking puzzle piece by piece. A host of small details play a role in why you continue to smoke. These little pieces of the puzzle are worth a careful look. Suddenly, everything will come together to form a large new picture. All you really want is a bit of advice and a quick recipe for quitting? Then it could very well be that you stop smoking quickly, but very soon you would be drawn back in again by one of your habitual thinking patterns. Faster than you realize, you will be holding a lit cigarette between your fingers. I know what I am talking about! Trust me. Understand what it is all about before you act.

*If you know your enemies and know yourself, you
will not be imperiled in a hundred battles.*
Sun Tzu, *The Art of War*

How the 30-Day Internet Program Works

The Internet program is your personal, practical guide. As a
reader you can log in for free for the first 10 days of the program
before you stop.

Login and Password!
Register at: www.my30dayquitsmokingcoach.com
Login name: Please page 294.
Password: Please page 294.

The First 10 Units Prepare You to Quit Smoking

It is here that you note what you do not like about smoking, why
you want to quit, how motivated you are, what you learned from
previous attempts to quit, what frightens you most about quitting,
and what is preventing you from quitting. You will also find a
cigarette-money counter and an addiction test. This will help you
make a decision and set a date for quitting. I would like to empha-
size that these are 10 units and not 10 days, as every smoker
needs to read the book and follow the Internet program at his or
her own pace to come to a decision. Setting a straitjacket of 10
days, which would also contain the date to quit smoking, would
not make sense. All it would do is create unnecessary pressure.
Although I recommend reading this book quickly, take as long as
you need to digest its preliminary information. Follow the 10
units of your program until you feel that the decision to quit is
good and correct for you. Only then do you set a date for quitting
that suits you and will make a success of it.

The Premium Program—Support for 20 Days After Quitting

Here you will receive daily support and motivation on how to succeed. There are 2 antirelapse trainings. You can track your success of being smoke-free day by day. Fitness and mood tests motivate you to see your improvements. You can download quit-smoking hypnosis sessions that will help you stay focused. Meet and talk to other smokers in the forum. You can learn more about how to cope with stress and train to resist smoking triggers. You also get daily nutrition tips. The topics range from nutrition for your nerves to keeping your weight down.

I Know You Like to Smoke

But You Can Quit—Now

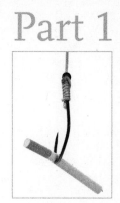

Part 1

Do You "Like" to Smoke?

1

From "Liking" to "Having" to Smoke

Just How Much Do You "Enjoy" Smoking?

You have a long and stressful day behind you and you want a treat. A cigarette . . . *flick* . . . what could be better than that? That feeling of pleasure as you inhale the smoke. A little cloud rises quietly up into the sky. And for a moment, the pace of the world is slower and more enjoyable. We smoke to relax. We smoke when we are stressed. We take time out. We smoke after a meal—one more thing to savor. The occasions are many.

So, why shouldn't your children also have some enjoyment? A cigarette to rid themselves of a hard, stressful day at school or when a friend goes off with their girlfriend. Lighting up will help them to get over that lousy feeling. Growing up is tough enough. And without cigarettes, all the stress and the roller coaster of emotions are really hard to take. Even just waiting for the school bus in the morning or for an irritating parent who was supposed to pick them up on time—even all that's a lot easier to take with a cigarette. What's pocket money for, anyway, if not for allowing yourself a treat?

But this is where the film "I enjoy smoking" begins to stall. After smokers have listed for me every conceivable advantage of smoking, they have to wince when I ask them whether they've encouraged their children to smoke.

Why does a smoker constantly go on and on about "enjoying" smoking? I am one of those people who never felt the need to justify the way they live. But as a smoker, I did just that. As time passed, it became increasingly clear to me that I was probably ticking off the advantages of smoking to convince myself that it was okay.

Smoking is a really tricky "habit." If we don't smoke, we want it more than anything, and then when we do smoke, we would rather not have to—yet we still believe we are smoking for the pleasure of it. And, although we "enjoy" it, we still don't want to recommend that anyone else start—especially anyone of an age at which we may ourselves have started—and would rather quit at some point.

Your First Cigarette

Can you still remember when you smoked your first cigarette? Did you smoke one with a friend or were you one of those people who had their first cigarette alone, just to try it out, so that later they could look like cool, experienced smokers? Do you remember feeling as if you were going to cough up your lungs after the first drag? Those dry, pungent fumes—disgusting! You felt queasy, sick, and dizzy, gasping for air as your bronchial tubes retracted and wanting to cough out the smoke as quickly as possible. A normal reaction. Smoke is always dangerous. We've been programmed by our instincts for millions of years to avoid inhaling toxic fumes.

Today, our children cough somewhat less from cigarettes than we did 20 years ago. How come? The cigarette industry has mixed a pile of substances into the tobacco to extend and calm the bronchial tubes, mildly sedate the windpipe, and make the smoke taste fresher. Why? Children and adolescents are the most important target group of that industry. Only 5% of smokers start to smoke after the age of 21, and often these just turn into social or occasional smokers. What does that mean for the industry? It means that the target group has to be captured as early on as possible. It's not only that young people are more easily influenced, but also that young brains are more easily altered and become addicted to nicotine significantly faster. Even after only a few cigarettes, the initial changes can be identified in the brain. And for a higher turnover and more profit, the industry needs many, many more up-and-coming nicotine recruits, because—put yourself in the shoes of the tobacco industry—the best customers die too early and the others decide to quit for some silly reason or another.

At Last, We Are Part of the Club

Back to your first cigarette. Every young person wants to be a part of the adult world, part of the clique of cool, young people who are in far better shape than their pimpled peers with their dental braces. Not to mention those embarrassing moments at the nightclub—now with a cigarette between our fingers, we had something cool to hold on to—when the second expensive drink was empty, the counter of the bar was packed to the gills, and we couldn´t lounge there on our elbows. Or when we felt someone was eyeing us or when an attractive stranger rendered us speechless—before uttering a load of gibberish, we could offer a cigarette and save the situation. Now that was cool.

Do you remember your first drags on a cigarette? First, we

6

had to practice hard to be able to inhale the harsh smoke and blow it out without coughing. Then came the elegant mastery of the cigarette and lighter, and developing the impressive way we blew smoke out of the side of our mouth without losing sight of that attractive-looking one. So, at last, we had joined the club and were a smoker!

We had seen plenty of this beforehand in films and television shows. In 70% of all US movies, somebody is smoking. Our screen idols smoke when getting to know each other, when trying to concentrate in tough situations, when relaxing after sex, at a bar, and on any other occasion we might care to imagine. So what could be so bad about it, when those whom we worship on-screen show us how normal smoking is?

The Curse of Normality

The secret of the cigarette as a drug is that when we start smoking, it tastes horrible. Nobody can imagine getting hooked on this disgusting smoke. Even the simple act of holding the cigarette gets on our nerves. A new recruit holds it far enough away to avoid the smoke's going up his or her nose. We take the "obligatory puffs," subjecting ourselves 5 or 6 times to the obnoxious-smelling smoke. Not exactly enjoyment. But we want to be part of the club from the outset. Or we let the cigarette burn away unobtrusively, all the while looking really cool. Not a hint of enjoyment during the first cigarettes we ever smoked.

Those who feel good after the first cigarette are few and far between. Stimulated, high, in a better mood—there is nothing of the sort. Perhaps we experience a little strange feeling in the head. So, let's compare the effects of smoking with the effects of other drugs.

Alcohol decreases inhibition, makes us jolly and more sociable, and renders it easier to make a pass at a girl. The cheap party drug ecstasy leads to the intense release of serotonin, a transmitter of happiness, giving us the feeling of being happy, cheerful, and satisfied. It makes people feel closer to one another and blurs the borders between us and thousands of others—the uninhibited feeling of raves is something very special. Marijuana relaxes us, gets us high, and we feel as if everything is easy. Everyone feels at their best on weed. Cocaine, on the other hand, stimulates the nervous system and makes thoughts and ideas just flow from the brain, while every feeling is amplified. But what about the first cigarettes we smoke, compared to these other drugs? They do nothing. For those just starting to smoke, nicotine is a total loser of a drug. At first, we feel like shit and nauseated. And on top of that, we have to practice. Nobody in their right mind would ever consider becoming dependent on this as a normal feeling. Then, there is the nasty taste. And on top of all that, nicotine does not even whisk us out of reality. "Impossible to ever become addicted to that," we said to ourselves.

Compared to other drugs, nicotine is neither enjoyable at the start, nor does it free us from our inhibitions or get us stoned. It is a purely social device: to be part of a group, to feel adult, and to look cool. And that is precisely what makes nicotine so cunning.

The Rapid Modification of the Nervous System

"But at some point, cigarettes started to taste good to me. I like to smoke now and find it satisfying. I've no idea why, but I feel more relaxed, calmer, and more alert after a cigarette."

Emotions are first created by chemical messengers—neurotransmitters—in the brain. Nicotine stimulates the release of dopamine, as well as other neurotransmitters. At first, this sounds like a benefit, but this release is quite minimal. The healthy nervous system of a novice smoker doesn't see this as a

8

great plus, as an advantage, or even as enjoyable, as compared with many other drugs. The little kick to the head with the accompanying, slightly woozy short-term feeling is hardly worth mentioning. Nevertheless, under the influence of nicotine, the nervous system is quickly modified, as early as after the first cigarette! At the spot where the nicotine docks onto the receptor, causing a small release of neurotransmitters (chemical messengers), the receptors become somewhat less sensitive. So it becomes just a bit more difficult for the body's own substances to stimulate sufficient amounts of these happiness neurotransmitters to achieve the same effect as nicotine.

Now, from time to time, you simply smoke another cigarette to help adjust your feeling of satisfaction a bit. Before you light up, you feel vaguely uncomfortable, without quite knowing why. You begin to "like" to smoke in order to feel normal again, even though you hardly notice it because you are too busy seeking acceptance of your peers and being cool.

Smoking Only Becomes Satisfactory Due to the Restructuring of the Brain

After a few cigarettes, the growing, young brain adapts to the effects of nicotine. Soon you notice the first symptoms of dependence.[2] Gradually, the nervous system is modified, and consequently, cigarettes become more and more satisfying. This change takes place at lightning speed. (I will show you just how fast in chapter 9.) The dark secret of the cigarette lies in these subtle changes to the nervous system: Nicotine works in a positive and rewarding way only when the nervous system has been altered so much that we feel a slight lack of neurotransmitters—a little dissatisfaction—which we then compensate with nicotine. Although nicotine offers little benefit or enjoyment for the beginner, it feels like an agreeable method of support once the nervous system is altered. Gradually we begin to "like" smoking, to like this tiny little boost into feeling like ourselves again—a feeling that we previously had naturally and for free without nicotine.

Nicotine: A Hard Drug?

The biggest ambush of cigarettes is that, due to the initial lack of any perceived "drug" effect from them, we don't actually see nicotine as an addictive drug. In our youthful exuberance, we are 100% sure that we cannot get addicted to this minimal effect, as had our dumb parents or older smokers who *have* to smoke.

It's only the modification of the brain that makes smoking satisfactory. This ambush makes nicotine a hard drug, the most addictive of all drugs. 38% of all beginner smokers (youths and adults) become addicted to nicotine and "happily" smoke for the next 10 to 20 years. In contrast, people experimenting with the following drugs become dependent at a lower rate: 23% become heroin dependent; 17%, cocaine dependent; 15%, alcohol dependent; and 9%, marijuana dependent. Children and adolescents are more likely than beginner adults to become nicotine dependent: fully 75% of all young smokers continue to smoke as adults.[3] The National Survey on Drug Use and Health estimates that each day, over 4,000 people under the age of 18 try their first cigarette. This amounts to more than 730,000 new smokers each year. Children and adolescents consume more than 1 billion packs of cigarettes every year.

"Hard" and "soft" drugs are only categories of public perception. If we were to compare nicotine with heroin in terms of their addiction potential and the time it takes to become addicted to them, then cigarettes rank first; likewise, tobacco is first among all other hard drugs. In addition, no other hard drug is the cause of so many deaths. 5 million people die annually from the effects of cigarette smoking, 443,000 in the United States alone. Annually. Any other drug fires at least one warning shot. People know that when they are on drugs, it's not a normal state of mind and that they cannot live and work permanently in such a state. But no one ever exalts the intoxicating effect of a cigarette. Instead, smokers just have the feeling that, after a few packs of the drug, they somehow feel better and enjoy it. Because this little pleasure feels so innocent and normal, it takes a long time until it becomes clear to smokers that they have long since become dependent on cigarettes and can no longer get through the day without them.

Would You Start Smoking Again?

Of course, we didn't know that after we first practiced smoking with a couple of cigarettes, that we would have to continue to smoke for the rest of our lives. If you could go back now, after a 10- to 20-year smoking career and be free to decide whether you would smoke that first cigarette again, what would you do?

- ❏ "I would start again. And I'm not sorry about it." Okay. You've had a good time smoking. But perhaps you want to start a new chapter in life anyway. You are still undecided. I don't want to talk you into anything. That never works. But nothing should stop you from having a look around in this book.
- ❏ "It would've been better if I'd never started. But back then, I was too stupid to say no." Almost certainly you were not too stupid. The advertising of the cigarette industry was so refined, movies and television manipulated you so subtly and continue to do so to this day, and the social pressure to fit in was so strong!

❏ "Yes, darn it. If I could make the decision again, I
wouldn't fall for it again." You seem to be fed up with
smoking. We just have to figure out how you can take
the leap.

When Did You First "Want to" Smoke?

Whereas you probably remember your first cigarette or even the
brand that you bought for the first time, very few smokers
remember when they first had the feeling that they "liked" to
smoke. When and how often have you bummed a cigarette,
because all of a sudden you "felt" like smoking? There's this
point when you no longer simply joined in smoking, but "liked" to
smoke. This is so subtle that you probably didn't even notice it.

The next step: Do you remember when you absolutely
"wanted" to buy a pack for the first time? Probably not. Because
this "wanting" is initially interpreted like this: "Oh, a cigarette
makes me feel good. There's smoking everywhere. So, I don't
have to think anything of the fact that I also enjoy smoking."
Over time, your brain became more and more trained to "like"
smoking in additional situations, to not only wheedle new doses
of nicotine but steadily increase the dosage. But at this stage,
because you viewed smoking as pleasurable, you probably didn't
notice how often you lit up.

It often takes years before you start thinking as a young adult
about the fact that you may like it "too much." Sex, drugs, and
rock and roll keep youth occupied. There's hardly any time to
think about more in your life.

Some 100,000 Hits Later

Can you remember the first time you ran out of cigarettes and
absolutely wanted to smoke *now*, or panicked because there were

no cigarettes in the house and the only gas station open was miles away? You probably don't remember. For a long time, your nervous system has been altered so effectively and you've been so deep in the nicotine trap for so long that the urge to smoke seems to be a natural drive. You've lost control over it. You no longer "enjoy" smoking but *need* to smoke. How did this happen?

At 20 cigarettes per day and 10 hits per cigarette, you flood your brain with 73,000 nicotine hits per year. After just 7 seconds, the nicotine in a lit cigarette has reached the receptors in the brain. The more you smoke, the more these receptors become accustomed to the flood of nicotine, become blunted, and require more and more nicotine to establish a basic sense of satisfaction.

Only gradually—after another 50,000 to 100,000 hits per year—does it dawn on smokers that it is as if they are remote-controlled. Suddenly, so many situations are no longer fun without a cigarette. Good things, such as a nice meal, are miserable without a cigarette. You have programmed your brain perfectly with thousands of conditioned hits that innumerable situations now require a cigarette: with your coffee, while waiting, after eating, before boarding a train, after disembarking, during a break, after work, with friends, with a beer, on the phone, after sex, in particular places, or when you smell others' smoke. How automatically, without thinking about it, do you grab a cigarette and call it a "habit"?

Another 100,000 Hits Later and You Smoke to Deal with the Stress

And then? Above all, boredom and stress are increasingly becoming smoking cues. You now need nicotine to calm your nerves. You barely notice that it is now the nicotine itself that stresses your whole body—for example, by releasing adrenaline or speeding up your heartbeat. The short-term relief of a cigarette stands in the foreground.

How did you cope at all in school when the teacher gave you a bad mark? Unbelievable, how tough you were without a cigarette as a child. No smoker would ever consider that smoking makes you tired as cigarettes seem to give a boost of energy. However, smokers also believe cigarettes have a calming effect. 2 opposite effects with one and the same drug?

Look reality in the eye: No child or nonsmoker ever needs a cigarette to feel better. Social pressure and the desire to fit in are the only reasons to *start* smoking, not to continue it. Also, you never needed cigarettes until you had smoked through your first pack, the sensitivity of your receptors was lowered, and then suddenly you started to "like" to smoke to correct this deficiency. Now cigarettes have become a necessary means of relief of negative feelings.

How Much Do You "Like" to Smoke?

First, you "liked" to smoke. Some 100,000 hits later, you are "driven by your likes." Now, you may already be at the point— after a smoking career of 10 to 20 years, or 730,000 to 2 million hits—where, with a guilty conscience and noticeable health issues, you are forced to "like" smoking. Many chain smokers have long left behind the "liking" and have no illusions about the addiction anymore. They surrender to their fate, because one simply has to do it. "I can't get away from it. I smoke. Discussion over."

The longer you smoke, the more the "liking" decreases and the "have to" increases. Then most smokers reach the point when they want to quit. You know best what stage of "liking" you're in. 30% of all smokers "like to" smoke so much that they try to quit once a year, but then still "like it too much" to actually break away from nicotine.

"Hurrah, I Smoke"

If you are convinced that you really smoke for pleasure, there's really no reason to stop. On the other hand, have you ever thought while buying a pack of cigarettes, "It's fantastic that I've started smoking, because otherwise I would have missed all this . . .?" Honestly, I've never heard this phrase from a smoker, because almost all smokers would actually prefer to be nonsmokers. And those who have stopped and then started again tell a story that almost always ends like this: ". . . unfortunately, then I smoked another one."

All smokers envy casual smokers who manage to only smoke a few cigarettes per day without giving it another thought. Only 10% of all smokers actually belong to this group. "5 cigarettes per day: That would be ideal!" Not at all. If you, as the average smoker, cut down the number of cigarettes, you would use a tremendous amount of energy simply to maintain this low level of smoking. The basic rule is: If you are addicted, you want to smoke more, not less. So smokers who merely cut back suffer the whole day, mostly for health reasons, until they can finally have their "one treat." These self-imposed "casual smokers" never tell me, "Hurrah, I smoke so little. That's a great feeling."

Is Smoking a Habit?

Most smokers speak of their desire for cigarettes as a "habit." Smoking is not a habit, the way eating certain foods is. Habits can be stopped at any time. When I drive in England on the left side of the road instead of on the right side as we do here, I turn off the old habit within a few seconds, as soon as I drive away from the airport in the rental car. It takes a little longer to not constantly confuse the turn signals and windshield wipers, which are also reversed on the steering wheel. But after a few initial blunders, I succeed at this as well. I simply switch habits without problems. I've also never gotten anxious and nervous or been close to having a panic attack because I could not drive on the right side. I also don´t get up at night to do a lap on the right side when the streets are empty. Why must we as smokers always speak of a "habit"? Habit and addiction are 2 completely different things.

Are You a Creature of Habit?

Creature of habit. That sounds as if I maintain my smoking habit according to some biological clock. Do you really want to describe yourself like that? What's left of your youthful high spirits, to not *have* to do anything? Were smokers not once the young people who rebelled against the adults? No one really likes to describe him- or herself as a petty-minded creature of habit. And what kind of habit would smoking be? Pumping 4,000 highly toxic substances into your lungs so you can die 10 to 15 years earlier than you otherwise would? I don't think that you would choose to develop such a "habit," if it were just a habit.

Do You Like to Eat Broccoli?

I really love to eat broccoli. Nevertheless, I cannot eat it 20 times a day. I do not bring broccoli with me on the road to nibble on, to increase my blood-broccoli levels. I won't become nervous and out of sorts if I cannot get it. I've also never needed to justify to other people why I love to eat broccoli. And I can stop eating broccoli anytime I want. It's the same with habits. You can get tired of even the best habits. Constantly eating broccoli can become boring; *needing* to eat it would be a nightmare. But with cigarettes, you can rarely get enough. Even after hundreds of thousands of nicotine hits, you still want more.

Did You Start Smoking Voluntarily?

"Of course, it was my decision." Yes, you decided to join in by smoking a few cigarettes. But did you also decide to continue smoking for a lifetime? It happened very gradually, progressing from just trying it out, to "enjoying" smoking, and later to "having to" smoke. When you began, you never anticipated getting hooked. You did not choose to make smoking a forced habit. All you did, with your very first cigarette, was learn how to handle and smoke it, not worrying about whether nicotine is addictive. After all, before a 1994 US inquiry into the psychoactive qualities of nicotine, the top executives of the tobacco industry swore under oath that nicotine was not addictive. You can actually see this oath by the CEOs of the 7 largest tobacco companies on YouTube. Just type in "Nicotine is not addictive."

It is fairly certain that as a teenager you never really thought about becoming dependent upon this substance or made a conscious choice to do this.

What even drives us to inhale acrid, pungent smoke? That is the great trick of the cigarette: We think we can stop at any time, because the smoke is not very pleasant and in the beginning we do it for social reasons. But then once we start to "like" smoking, we stop noticing that we don't really like it at all.

Why Are Cigarettes So Widely Accepted?

Cigarettes are a hard drug—they are extremely addictive, and more people die yearly of them than with any other drug. Why is it, then, that cigarettes are so accepted? The answer is relatively simple. A heroin addict or alcoholic cannot work, or only partially. In addition, these drugs have a hallucinogenic effect; they are intoxicating. They lead to the loss of control and misbehavior, because the threshold of social awareness drops or people slide into existential nothingness, as can happen with crack or heroine. Physical deterioration sets in very quickly. In contrast, the tobacco smoker remains completely normal, is able to work, and doesn't die for another 20 to 30 years.

But let me modify that: In terms of behavior, mood, and ability to function, smokers are no different from nonsmokers . . . as long as they have enough nicotine in their blood. Only when the nicotine level drops do they have to face restlessness, nervousness, irritability, and a lack of concentration. But every smoker avoids this by simply smoking another cigarette. In that light, cigarettes are seen as the petty bourgeois of all drugs and are accepted as normal. The dubious distinction of the tobacco industry is that it has made smoking socially acceptable as a so-called habit, and has thereby concealed the dangers of smoking and addiction.

"Nevertheless, I Am a Habitual Smoker"

Let's say you smoke after eating, with friends, or to relax. Okay. If you are a habitual smoker, then it probably will not be hard to stop this habit. Let's do a test: Throw away your cigarettes! *Now*! Nothing forces you to smoke them. It's like liking broccoli. If in the next week you don't once become restless or nervous and don't feel like you have to smoke, then you needn't read the rest of this book.

However, after only a short time, you probably will have this restless, empty feeling that something is missing. This can grow into fear and panic. The thought "I need a cigarette" is now compulsive. This has nothing to do with habit.

Unmask Why You "Enjoy" Smoking

18

We've already seen how little many smokers, in fact, "like" to smoke. Most smokers actually have no idea why they smoke. They just do it. It comes and goes like a hungry feeling, and after they've smoked it goes away again. The important thing is this: Without understanding why you "enjoy" smoking, you'll never be able to really quit. You'll constantly have the feeling that you are "doing without" something.

Many methods to quit smoking only focus on the fact that smoking ruins your health, that it may take away on average 5 to 8 years from your life, and that the privilege of smoking costs a fortune. Nonsmokers and doctors will try to get you to quit by telling you why you should not smoke. Only none of this works: You will find it hard to quit if you focus on these arguments to stop smoking—*because you do not smoke for the reasons that they say you should not smoke!* Otherwise, most smokers would have quit a long time ago. If this were so, there would probably be no more smokers anymore.

We "like" to smoke for quite different reasons: for pleasure, from desire, to reduce stress, to feel calmer or more concentrated. To quit, you have to work on addressing *these* reasons. Only when you have unmasked the "liking," will you get rid of cigarettes easily.

Give yourself a tap on the shoulder. You've managed the first chapter. Even if the drug wanted to stop you, you have prevailed.

THE BOTTOM LINE

▸ Smoking is a social device: One starts in order to fit in, to be cool, and to seem grown-up.

- ► Nicotine is a hard drug and is more addictive than any other drug.
- ► The brain of adolescents is altered after just a few cigarettes.
- ► Only by nicotine's changing the brain's neurotransmitter system do cigarettes become satisfying. Only then do beginning smokers start to like smoking and then very quickly lose control.
- ► With nicotine, smokers achieve a small lift to the "normal level" of nonsmokers or to how they felt before they became a smoker.
- ► Smoking is not a habit, it is an addiction.
- ► Although you decided to smoke a few cigarettes as a teenager, it was not your choice to continue to smoke for a lifetime.
- ► It is difficult to quit based on the reasons that tell you why you should not smoke. Only when you understand why you "like" and "enjoy" smoking will you be able to stop easily, because then you will know that you won´t miss out on anything.

2

Advertisements and Hollywood as Role Models

IN A HURRY TO QUIT SMOKING? Then you could skip this chapter. (But which smoker has ever been in a hurry to quit? Most would prefer to postpone the scary moment of the "last cigarette" for just a little longer. With this in mind, you might as well continue reading.) This chapter is about the way we see ourselves as smokers and how this is influenced by advertising and Hollywood. The nicotine industry in Germany spends 390 million euros per year on brainwashing advertisements that focus on young people—and experts believe that many billions of dollars were being pushed over the tables in Hollywood.

When you started smoking, there were probably still newspaper ads and TV and radio commercials that promoted it. Today this kind of advertising is banned; however, the total advertising budget has remained the same over the past 10 years in Germany, where nowadays, the money is pumped into sports sponsorship, music events, billboards, and cinema advertising, or it is spent on promotion in clubs, where samples of cigarettes are used to lure young people.

The nicotine industry remains interested in young people because they are easily influenced and young brains become very quickly addicted. 9 out of 10 smokers start before they are 21 years old. The average starting age is 11 to 14 years. Millions of dollars are still used profitably on more subtle, subliminal means of advertising, to make young people nicotine-dependent as quickly as possible.

Did You Decide to Smoke?

"Of course, it was my decision to smoke." We all say this as long as we smoke. But let's take a closer look.

You probably know the brand obsession children have, such as for certain sneakers. It absolutely has to be that specific cool brand; no others will do. Even T-shirts must bear the "right" logo; otherwise a crisis might happen. The advertising industry exploits the enormous receptivity and suggestibility of children and adolescents by imprinting on their brain the desire for par-ticular products. This is called branding in the language of advertising; it hails literally from the verb *to brand*, as is done with cattle. An example: In one survey, 30% of 3-year-olds and 91% of 6-year-olds who were interviewed in the United States could, after seeing the Camel-campaign cartoon, associate the logo with the brand. At the beginning of this Camel campaign, 0.5% of young people smoked Camels. 3 years later, it was 32.8% of young people.

Brands are a form of identification and express a particular lifestyle that can be demonstrated by them. The ads never actu-ally show children or teenagers smoking, but cunningly pro-vide attractive adult role models for them to emulate. Young people in search of role models are awed and bound with billions of dollars to a particular cigarette brand: the open-minded Lucky Strike smoker, the independent Gauloise type, the freedom- and adventure-loving Marlboro type, or the elegant, high-society John Player Special smoker. Young smokers' cigarette brands become a symbol of how they want themselves to be perceived in future, the image they want to portray of themselves. This advertising imagery remains active even in adults. Loyalty to one's own cigarette brand is extremely high and well branded.

When thinking of role models, just look at Formula 1 and its most famous driver, Michael Schumacher, in his red Marlboro Ferrari suit. For young smokers, this has a magical attraction. Schumacher would never smoke, of course, because that would permanently decrease the oxygen supply to his brain and his concentration. But advertising links things in your head, things that have absolutely nothing to do with each other.

One only has to entice children and teenagers to try cigarettes of a certain brand, and because the physiological changes that addict the young brain set in after just a few cigarettes, the objective is quickly achieved: they will soon be caught in the nicotine trap for long-term business. Approximately 140,000 children and teenagers in Germany are recruited annually as "replacement smokers," as the nicotine industry calls them in marketing terms. This is why the advertising budget of the tobacco industry was targeted mainly at young smokers. According to the documents of R. J. Reynolds: "Younger smokers are the only source of replacement smokers [. . .] only 5% start after the age of 24."[4] Another internal document says: "CAMEL FILTER, the brand, must increase its share penetration among the 14–24 age group [. . .] which represent tomorrow's cigarette business . . ."[5] In contrast, adult smokers do not need advertising—from the point of view of the industry they are already addicted, and even without the advertising continue to buy their preferred product with high brand loyalty. It is rare for adult smokers to be enticed by advertising to switch brands even though in blind tests only 5% of all smokers can even identify their brand.

Were You Also Lured into the Nicotine Trap by Advertising?

As a smoker, you always think that you chose to smoke. But how strong were the advertisement images, the entertainment media and social pressures, to try your first cigarettes and thereby get caught in the nicotine trap? This has less to do with your own decision than you think.

Sample packs are an example of how addiction can be effectively marketed. In Germany, at club events with special DJs and music, nice girls and boys distribute lighters or replace half-empty cigarette packs with full ones. Of course, the tobacco dealers insist that these actions are exclusively directed toward adults. One can also participate there in contests, where it is stated in the fine print that the participant must be over 18 years old. Studies show that the distribution of sample packages can increase new smokers by up to twenty-twofold, because the addiction sets in extremely quickly.[6] The targeted placement of billboards and neon signs at bus stops in the vicinity of schools is also very popular. Germany is the only country in the EU that has not yet banned billboard and cinema advertising of tobacco products. But there are strong "self-restrictions" of the tobacco industry. In the cinema, for example, cigarette advertisements may indeed be shown, but only after 6 p.m. by which time, of course, adolescents have gone to bed . . . (!). Most of these advertising forms and promotional instruments were still allowed when you started smoking. In the third world, such traps for young smokers are still allowed and the major growth for the tobacco dealers is in these markets.

Images in Advertising That You Cannot Get Out Of Your Head

How many of the images and personality concepts promoted by advertising at the time when you began to smoke, do you still have in your head today? Why do you smoke a particular brand, for example, if you're not supposed to have been influenced by the advertising? Even though the images about a certain lifestyle, enjoyment, and freedom recede rapidly behind the addiction, they remain active in your subconscious as a justification for smoking.

Are you sure you decided to smoke without external influences, just because from the very beginning it gave you such enjoyment? Or did you want to try it just once, because you wanted to be cool and grown-up and the advertising conveyed this feeling to you? And did you plan then on continuing to smoke that brand throughout your entire life? Were you really not at all influenced by the images in advertising? If you answered no to all of the questions above, I—if I were a tobacco company—would be bitterly disappointed. But the nicotine dealers hooked you anyway. That's what counts. You have been a great source of revenue for them.

Hollywood Does Most of the Shaping

Films and television have an even greater impact on smokers than do other marketing strategies. A suave, smoking Sharon Stone or Leonardo DiCaprio, or the slim and emancipated sex and fashion icon Sarah Jessica Parker—who puffed away every week on the TV series *Sex and the City*—have been important role models, especially for the young beginner smokers. Even in typical US television series about hospitals, you see doctors smoking. What could more clearly convey to teenagers that smoking cannot be that bad for their health? Even in Tom & Jerry and other cartoons, there is smoking.

Check this out: Here is an excerpt from the list of the top smoking actresses.[7] In fact, most of them smoke only in the movies, not in their private lives, because you age faster if you smoke. And this would be bad for their careers. So in how many movies did these actors smoke?

25

Sarah Jessica Parker in 45 films, Catherine Deneuve in 41, Bette Davis in 37, Holly Hunter in 35, Melanie Griffith in 28, Joan Crawford in 27, Joan Collins in 26, Romy Schneider in 26, Isabelle Huppert in 25, Susan Sarandon in 23, Marlene Dietrich in 23, Jeanne Moreau in 21, Kirstie Alley in 21, Lana Turner in 19, Kim Cattrall in 19, Ava Gardner in 18, Shirley MacLaine in 18, Ginger Rogers in 18, Rita Hayworth in 18, Jane Fonda in 17, Jacqueline Bisset in 17, Jessica Lange in 17, Anita Ekberg in 16, Sharon Stone in 16, Anne Bancroft in 16, Juliette Binoche in 15, Faye Dunaway in 15, Diane Keaton in 14, Elizabeth Taylor in 14, Simone Signoret in 14, Penélope Cruz in 13, Winona Ryder in 13, Lauren Bacall in 13, Sophia Loren in 13, Demi Moore in 13, Franka Potente in 13, Meryl Streep in 13, Goldie Hawn in 13, Brigitte Bardot in 13, Sigourney Weaver in 13, Nicole Kidman in 13, Heike Makatsch in 13, Kate Blanchet in 12, Gwyneth Paltrow in 12, Gena Rowlands in 12, Senta Berger in 12, Julie Christie in 12, Drew Barrymore in 11, Sandra Bullock in 11, Vanessa Redgrave in 11, Michelle Pfeiffer in 11, Kate Winslet in 11, Whoopi Goldberg in 11, Meg Ryan in 11, Bette Midler in 11, Angelina Jolie in 11, Madonna in 11, Sophie Marceau in 11, Greta Garbo in 10, Elke Sommer in 10, Uma Thurman in 10, Cameron Diaz in 10 . . .

An analysis of the 250 highest-grossing movies of the last 10 years reveals the following: 85% of them contain smoking scenes; in 28%, a tobacco brand is shown.[8] In one third of all films directed specifically at teenagers, cigarette brands are clearly visible. The advantage of US movies is the fact that they can be seen worldwide. Although the tobacco companies have formally pledged not to use product placement, 80% of the packs shown were of 4 major cigarette brands. A single brand, Marlboro, accounted for 40%. In fact, within the last 10 years, the number of actors who show their cigarette brands on camera has increased tenfold.

"Surely this happens by accident . . . sure, some cigarette packs were simply on the set and the camera just zoomed on them by chance." The nicotine mafia claims it does not support Hollywood. However, an analysis of the internal documents of the tobacco industry shows exactly what smoking actors were being paid, as well as the costs for each product's placement in shows and movies.[9] Like actual smokers, smoking actors are not puffing away purely because they "enjoy" it.

How Strongly Films Influence "Wanting to Try"

Celebrities with whom we identify exert a big influence on our unconscious. 60% of the leading actors smoke in US films today—more than in the 1950s. How much does the media manipulate today's young people?

Surveys have shown that when their favorite star smoked in a TV series, young people started to smoke more often than did those whose favorite star was a nonsmoker. In a German study, 5,585 children and young adults were asked about their smoking habits and their knowledge of more than 400 movies.[10] There was smoking in three quarters of these films. Children who had seen most of the films had tried smoking twice as often as had children who had seen only a few of the films. And in another study that interviewed 3,500 teenagers, the results are even more interesting: It turned out that the nonsmoking youths who could identify most of the smoking scenes from 50 popular films in which there was heavy smoking, were 3 times more likely to start smoking themselves one year later than were the ones who did not know these scenes.[11]

Studies or not, the rationale for this is clear when you think about it for a moment. How do we orient ourselves as teenagers and whom do we admire? TV characters almost feel like family. Movie stars are great role models. This is the best way to learn that smoking is a natural part of when you want to be cool, when you are thinking, when solving a difficult crime, when you are having relationship problems, when you are stressed, when you want to turn someone on to you or you are in bed afterward. Even those condemned to death are offered a final cigarette in films. This is not without effect on us. Even very young people whose family does not smoke are exposed to a variety of smoking situations by watching TV or movies, and learn how and when to smoke by emulating their favorite characters or stars.

Also, as adults, our smoking keeps being confirmed by the celebrities who smoke on-screen. It is inescapable. There is a constant brainwashing that is presented to us through our stars' smoking in different situations. Give it a try: For the next few days, pay particular attention to how many movies or television programs show people smoking, and in which situations. Although this will temporarily increase your desire to smoke, it should be an interesting experiment to look for the many ways in which smoking is a deliberate element of the entertainment industry.

Did You Consciously Decide to Smoke?

Probably not. Peer pressure, the billions that have been put into cigarette advertising and sponsorship, and above all, an overwhelmingly smoky film culture have demonstrated smoking behaviors thousands of times. We were not stupid but alert,

28

curious young people. Therefore we tried it. And it didn´t stay a habit. Very quickly we "liked" smoking. And then everything happened all by itself. The conviction that they have always "wanted to" smoke is part of the self-understanding of all smokers. But a closer look shows that most smokers did not really decide to start smoking; rather, they were lured into a trap with targeted advertising and calculated manipulation by Hollywood. Then the nicotine trap quickly snapped shut.

THE BOTTOM LINE

- ▶ Cigarette advertisements have focused on making children and young people try smoking.
- ▶ Movie and television stars who smoke on screen give an additional strong impulse and also provide the dependent smokers with strong role models.
- ▶ The rapid onset of addiction forces us to continue smoking because we're stuck in the nicotine trap.

3

How Nicotine Dealers Get You Hooked

NOBODY WOULD INHALE SMOKE IF IT didn't contain nicotine. Cigarettes are the most efficient form of nicotine delivery. That is why it was the strategic aim of the nicotine industry to increase the uptake and speed of nicotine delivery to the brain. The faster and stronger nicotine floods the brain, the quicker dependency arises—particularly in the case of young people. Nicotine is a unique customer retention program, bringing maximum profits.

Up until 1995, the internal research work of the nicotine industry was inaccessible. Only after the judgment in the case of *The State of Minnesota vs. the Tobacco Industry*, were millions of internal documents published on the Internet. These reveal:

- how the nicotine industry intentionally refined the addictive nature of tobacco
- how, despite better judgment, it was denied in public that nicotine was addictive

- how details of the toxic substances and nicotine content were manipulated
- how attempts were made to undermine the findings of independent research through well-sponsored research
- how children were made a long-term target group for addiction through aromatic improvements and additives designed to calm the bronchial tubes
- how politicians, journalists, and scientists were frequently bribed with consultant contracts

The nicotine dealers damaged intentionally and systematically the health of millions of Americans. The biggest tobacco companies reached an agreement with the attorney general to pay $206 billion (not million) to resolve all remaining US state claims over health costs related to smoking. That is a tiny amount compared to the profits of the nicotine dealers.

Addiction as a Commercial Target

The tobacco company R. J. Reynolds documented internally, "We are basically in the nicotine business [. . .] it is in the best long-term interest of RJR to be able to control and effectively utilize every pound of nicotine we purchase. Effective control of nicotine in our products should equate to a significant product performance and cost advantage."[12]

The issue here is not about enjoyment of a product, but about marketing addiction by making nicotine as bioavailable as possible.

Addiction keeps the tills ringing. Why, in the 1970s, did the Marlboro brand overtake Winston to become the leading cigarette brand sold in the USA? The answer lies in the ammonium technology that made Marlboro smokers more quickly and severely addicted. When ammonium is added, the nicotine is better absorbed (bioavailability) and floods the brain more rapidly. This is but one deceptive practice that emerges from internal documents of the nicotine industry.[13]

How People Are Made More Quickly Addicted to Nicotine

In the 1960s to '80s, the addictive potential of cigarettes was increased. The aims:

1. Nicotine intake should be increased and it should be absorbed more quickly.
2. Deeper inhalation to increase nicotine absorption should be combined with decreased irritation. This is how to gain more young recruits.

AMMONIUM: This can be used to change the pH value of the tobacco. The more basic, the better the nicotine is released. Nicotine reaches the brain receptors more quickly and gives a better kick. Having a quick kick is the core of most drugs and causes severe addiction. Internal research documents confirm that the nicotine industry has known this since 1962. The nicotine kick is the reason why one brand "tastes" better than another. Today, all nicotine dealers use ammonium technology.

As authorities and the public demanded cigarettes with lower nicotine content, the industry invented "light" cigarettes with an allegedly lower nicotine content. But in reality, the ammonium released significantly more nicotine and made it more bioavailable. This trick was uncovered only decades later. The nicotine dealers declared ammonium as a "taste-enhancing" additive, so as to gain approval from the authorities.

NOTE: Nicotine patches do not cause dependency because, in this case, the nicotine reaches the brain much more slowly. The drug kick accounting for dependency is missing.

SPECIAL FILTER SYSTEMS: Special filters enhanced removal of acid and the addition of chemical bases. The more basic the tobacco, the better bioavailability of the addictive nicotine.

(continued on pg 32)

32

(continued from previous page)

SUGAR: This sounds like an innocent additive. Acetaldehyde is produced by burning sugar; this accelerates and amplifies the addictive effect of nicotine.

COCOA: When cocoa burns, it becomes bromine and enlarges the bronchial tubes, so more nicotine can be inhaled more deeply. Licorice has the same effect.

LEVULINIC ACID: This substance takes the edge off the tobacco flavor and reinforces nicotine binding with the receptors in the brain by some 30%.

MENTHOL: Smoking must be made easier for smokers suffering from respiratory problems, so they will continue to smoke. Menthol reduces the sensation of irritation and pain in the respiratory tract, and calms the bronchial tubes and expands them. This results in deeper inhalation without any unpleasant feeling or burning sensation. Menthol also masks the pungent taste of tobacco smoke. The smoke feels cooler and fresher, an important point when wooing the youth market. All cigarette brands today make use of menthol additives even in normal cigarettes, as young "replacement smokers" are needed and inhalation must be made easy for them. In addition, menthol slows down the decomposition of nicotine, so the hit lasts longer.

LITTLE UNNOTICED NICOTINE INCREASES: US studies show that over the past 8 years, and unnoticed by most smokers, tobacco companies have increased the nicotine content of cigarettes by 11%.[14] This all but guarantees addiction, even among lighter smokers. Customer retention is king . . .

VARIOUS CHEMICALS SLOW DOWN THE SPEED OF BURNING: By slowing down the speed at which the tobacco burns, the smoker gets more puffs from every cigarette and has a higher intake of nicotine.

"LIGHT" CIGARETTES: This is the biggest trick in the game: The nicotine content on the packet is ascertained by smoking machines. But human smokers consume the same amount of nicotine and toxic substances from "light" cigarettes as they do from normal cigarettes.

Inside, a movie that stars Al Pacino and Russell Crowe, shows how a former head of research in a cigarette company uncovers scandalous practices of the tobacco companies and how he is stalked. A real thriller to watch.

The Scam of "Light" Cigarettes

Do you smoke "lights" or their successors, in their light blue or pastel-colored packets? You thought these would be healthier and would have less tar and nicotine? With "lights," the nicotine industry has deliberately deceived you.

During the 1970s, the tobacco industry lost an increasing number of smokers as awareness of the health risks grew. Lowering the addictive nicotine content was not an option, let alone a possibility. British American Tobacco (Lucky Strike, Gauloise, Pall Mall) stated in an internal note: "A cigarette that does not deliver nicotine cannot satisfy the habituated smoker and cannot lead to habituation, and would therefore almost certainly fail" and "Weaning the smoker away from nicotine habituation and depriving him of parts of the gratification desired or expected . . . may be equivalent to long term liquidation of the cigarette industry."[15] As they "could" not reduce the nicotine content, the cigarette companies came up with the idea of the "light" cigarette.

For almost 30 years, "lights" stopped many smokers from quitting, as they believed they had made a personal compromise to switch to cigarettes that were allegedly healthier and less damaging. A survey of 12,000 ex-smokers shows how profitable this must have been for the nicotine industry. Compared with regular smokers, only half as many smokers of "lights" quit, on account of switching instead to the so-called healthier "light" version.[16] The United States and EU have now banned terms such as "mild," "low tar," "light," "ultra light," and "ultra" from continuing to deceive the consumer.

The Smoking Machine Scam

"Light" cigarettes work as follows: Tiny holes are made in the filters so that additional air is inhaled. In this way, the tobacco seems somewhat milder for the smoker and can be inhaled more deeply.

For toxic substance analysis—which appears on the packet—cigarettes are tested in standardized smoking machines. (3 guesses who invented them!) The thin metal grippers do not cover the tiny pinholes in the filters through which the additional air is inhaled. As a result, the data of the analysis show extremely low nicotine and tar values. In some cases, even tobacco with a higher nicotine concentration could now be used and still show low nicotine content. With the smoking machine scam, nicotine dealers were able to print "officially" lower values on the packets of the supposedly healthier "light" cigarettes. Then millions were spent on "light" advertising campaigns to spread the joyous news.

But, of course, no one smokes by holding the cigarette with a pair of tweezers on pouted lips. Smokers hold the filter well between the lips and block the pinholes partly with their fingers. As a result, between 40% and 50% more nicotine and tar in "light" cigarettes enter the respiratory system than is measured by the machines.[17] Philip Morris has been aware of this since the so-called Lip Study in 1969. This was just one of the typical conjuring tricks of the drug mafia, which brought in billions of dollars for 30 years, until the ban on "light" cigarettes.

Light Smokers Inhale Toxic Substances More Deeply

Nicotine producers knew from early studies at the beginning
of the 1970s that, if the smoke is diluted with extra air, the
addicted smoker merely takes deeper and stronger puffs. Every
smoker's addicted brain knows quite precisely how much nicotine it requires to avoid withdrawal symptoms. "Lights" smokers puff more intensively and more frequently on each cigarette
to avoid nicotine withdrawal symptoms, or simply smoke more
"light" cigarettes to get the same cumulative hit. And so, without even realizing it, the "light" smoker achieves exactly the
same nicotine level as when previously smoking normal
cigarettes.

$150 Million in Damages for the "Light" Lie

Many lawsuits are still ongoing involving these lies. For example, a US court sentenced Philip Morris to pay $150 million in
damages, owing to deceit and negligence, to the heirs of a single
"light cigarettes" smoker who had died.

The ingenious invention of a "healthier, and safer" "light"
cigarette had deceived millions of health-conscious smokers,
many of whom were otherwise ready to quit. By keeping them
addicted to just as much nicotine as were they to smoke regular
cigarettes, the drug industry had an iron hold over them—but
with one difference, which was known since the beginning of
the 1970s: Deeper inhalation results in even more toxic substances getting deeper into the lung.[18] As a result, smokers of
"lights," who were tricked into inhaling more deeply, develop
different and more lethal types of cancer. They would have been
better off smoking normal cigarettes to get the nicotine they
needed. Today, the stance of British American Tobacco is the
following: "Light refers only to the aroma, nothing else."

The Tobacco Industry as Nicotine Dealer

In the past, the tobacco industry used advertising films with romantic images of tobacco being hung up to dry in the kiln by hand in a picturesque Virginia landscape to give the impression of tobacco as part of a cultural heritage.

And as you've just read, the nicotine producers pursued their optimization targets by all manner of devious means, from buying celebrity role models to entice you to smoke, to using additives to make as many people become addicted at as young an age as possible. Do you want to continue being manipulated like this? In your youth, did you really imagine you would have to smoke for the rest of your life because a drug industry had manipulated you?

"Nicotine Does Not Cause Addiction"

"Our industry is founded on the basis of designing, producing and selling attractive forms of nicotine dosages," was stated in tobacco industry internal documents dated 1972.[19] But the various patents, additives, and internal documents of these same nicotine dealers leave no room for doubt. Look at the statements of the chairmen of 7 boards of the largest tobacco companies, each lying in succession when under oath in 1994. The nicotine cartel closes ranks!

THE BOTTOM LINE

- ▶ You have been led to believe for decades that nicotine does not cause addiction.
- ▶ Various additives have been used to manipulate you and get you addicted quickly in your youth.
- ▶ Many smokers were prevented from quitting through the invention of the allegedly healthier "light" cigarette.

4

The Biochemistry
of Happiness

Measuring Enjoyment—How Is That Possible?

"It's not possible to measure the enjoyment and satisfaction I get from a cigarette. I simply enjoy smoking!" I believe you—I "enjoyed" it myself for well over 20 years, precisely that "enjoyment" you are feeling. But were you never amazed that some cigarettes "taste good" and that you enjoy them in particular, whereas others are pretty insignificant? And what is it that you are actually enjoying? Are you smoking because you have the choice, or is this "enjoyment" steered by an addicted brain?

As a matter of fact, enjoyment and satisfaction can be measured. In the following experiment, 4 smokers took part in 4 days of 6-hour smoking tests in which they had to assess how much they enjoyed smoking and how satisfied they felt with the last cigarette after 6 hours.[20]

ENJOYING SMOKING.

There is a direct correlation between nicotine deficit and the feeling of "enjoyment."

CIGARETTES WITHIN A 6-HOUR PERIOD	"ENJOYMENT" AND SATISFACTION	NUMBER OF CIGARETTE DRAGS
0 cigarettes: Only 1 cigarette was smoked after the 6-hour period.	**85%** "enjoyed smoking" and found it "satisfying." There is a clear indication of satisfaction from raising the nicotine level.	**15 DRAGS** were taken on average from 1 cigarette. Smokers wanted to suck the very last drop of nicotine from the cigarette they had yearned for after 6 hours.
2 cigarettes: 1 cigarette after 3 hours and the other after 6 hours	**71%** "enjoyed smoking" and found it "satisfying." In the experiment, after 3 hours, smokers still felt relief from another cigarette.	**14 DRAGS** on average were "enjoyed" by smokers.
5 cigarettes: 1 cigarette hourly	**68%** "enjoyed" smoking. The normal period between cigarettes is 1 hour, after which most smokers would "enjoy" a cigarette. That is why many end up smoking 12 to 20 per day.	**13 DRAGS:** For the majority of smokers, this was the average number. Take it easy! You don't have to smoke the filter!
11 cigarettes: 1 cigarette every 30 minutes	**48%** Only half said that the smoking experience was "satisfying" or that they had particularly "enjoyed" smoking. With a total of 11 cigarettes—1 every 30 minutes—the nicotine in the blood had reached a high level. Cigarettes no longer "tasted" particularly good.	**10 DRAGS:** "Okay. I'm a smoker." It isn't really necessary. Smoking had been more "enjoyable" in the past.

"Enjoying Smoking" Is Nothing More Than a Mechanism

The lower the level of nicotine in the body, the higher smokers assess their "enjoyment" of smoking—the level of pleasure and satisfaction. Smokers taking the test all had a similar behavior: The longer the period between cigarettes, the more frequent and deeper the drags, to get as much nicotine as possible from each cigarette. That is why there is little purpose in reducing the number of cigarettes by 2 or 3 per day. Smokers will simply try to get more nicotine from the other cigarettes, and on top of this, will inhale toxic substances even more deeply into their lungs, as when smoking "light" cigarettes.

Smokers tested showed quite clearly: Cigarettes are "enjoyed" most when the smoker has a greater nicotine deficit. That is, the enjoyment experienced is a direct consequence of your reduced nicotine level. You become a nicotine puppet. This is a far cry from the image of pleasure and way of life you have chosen and in the cigarette advertising you've seen.

If you like eating oysters, you take pleasure in them. You wouldn't like oysters better after 60 minutes simply because your oyster blood level is dropping. Quite the opposite: Eating additional oysters every hour would become torture. In talking about nicotine, we're not talking about a habit or a deliberate pleasure but, plain and simple, about nicotine levels and degradation times, withdrawal symptoms, the number and depth of nicotine inhalations, and a "satisfaction" that is nothing more than the reduction of withdrawal symptoms. Of course, you find satisfaction and pleasure in smoking your way out of a low nicotine level that is making you uncomfortable. As the nicotine level in the body is halved after 30 minutes, many smoke between 12 and 20 cigarettes daily, not to feel good but to allay repeatedly feeling bad.

Smoking by the Numbers—The Smoking Pattern

In the study we mentioned, 71% of smokers tested had a strong desire to smoke a cigarette after 6 hours; 49%, after 3 hours; and 28%, after 30 minutes.[21] There is nothing surprising about that for a smoker. The longer you wait, the more you want to smoke. So, why all these percentages? To make things complicated? No. "I feel like smoking" sounds like a wonderful feeling of freedom. In fact, the seemingly petty "I feel like a percentage" has nothing to do with adventure or freedom, but a simple automatic compulsion.

Three hours! For many that is the limit for feeling okay without a cigarette. I am sure you know the feeling. You are sitting in a restaurant with friends over a several-course meal. But even before the dessert arrives, you are standing outside, puffing away . . . of course, because you "want to" and because you "enjoy" it. Even the most delicious chocolate cake becomes a torture if you can't get out for a cigarette before the meal is over. This makes a misery of a wonderful meal, because you are dissatisfied when your nicotine level has gone low and you aren't permitted to smoke indoors. It has brought about one of the mini-stress situations which you as a smoker experience again and again throughout the day. And finally, whenever you can light up, you drag away with "enjoyment" on your cigarette.

This Is How Addiction Works

With 20 cigarettes puffed 10 times apiece, you flood your nervous system daily with 200 small doses of nicotine. After a few seconds, the nicotine is taken up by the many receptors in the body. Stress hormones are released. Heartbeat and blood pressure rise. After 7 seconds, the nicotine has reached the receptors in the brain. These receptors are located in the reward area and are made for substances produced by the body which stimulate the release of happiness transmitters. Nicotine causes structural changes to these receptors in 2 ways: Because of the frequent flooding of nicotine molecules, the receptors quickly become less sensitive in general and less sensitive for substances produced by the body as well. At the same time, nicotine increases the number of receptors. Addicted smokers have twice as many receptors as nonsmokers do. Both of these facts mean, unfortunately, that you need an ever-increasing amount of nicotine to produce the same effect, to stimulate the release of happiness transmitters. This is called habituation. You find the same effect with any drug. That is why the number of cigarettes you smoke daily increases over the years for you to reach a similarly satisfying effect and to feel half-normal. Internal marketing documents from the tobacco industry actually include this happy expectation of additional sales in the progressively increasing addictive nature of each smoker.[22] The number of cigarettes smoked daily increases on average by 30% over 10 to 15 years of smoking. Over the years, smokers spent more and more money to keep their receptors happy with the increasing habituation and addiction.

Smoking—Just to Feel Better

Like all drugs that permanently change the transmitter metabolism of the brain, the increased number of receptors also increases mood swings and susceptibility to stress. If you don't smoke, the receptors in the reward center of the brain remain unoccupied and the mood deteriorates. You become increasingly nervous, irritable, and unable to concentrate. Smokers have too many receptors in the brain for the body alone to produce sufficient amounts of the substance (acetylcholine) to occupy the receptors and get enough happiness transmitters. That is why you have to go on smoking nicotine to feel normal. So, unlike what many smokers think, smoking has no advantages: Smoking causes permanent structural changes and deficiencies in the brain's reward center, which can only be satisfied by more and more nicotine. You "enjoy smoking" because it relieves a bad feeling, an emptiness, a niggling feeling of dissatisfaction. The smoker experiences this relief as a reward or enjoyment. He or she feels better—just like any other drug addict who has gotten a fix. The need for a cigarette grows the lower your nicotine level drops and the less the receptors are occupied.

The only way to reverse the changes in your brain's reward system is to drop smoking for several weeks. Once your body is weaned off nicotine, the number of receptors decreases and they become sensitive again. Soon your nerve transmitters are sufficiently restored for you to begin to feel more satisfaction from them. Your mood stabilizes and you become less susceptible to stress. You again experience pleasure and enjoyment without needing a drug to do it for you.

How Boring Can a Drug Be?

When you smoke, you don't even get high; you have to compensate with nicotine for a bad feeling that is caused in the first place by nicotine, just to feel normal again. And you even pay for this. With each cigarette pack, you buy feeling normal—a feeling that every nonsmoker already has and that you had before you started smoking! From the video at the end of the chapter, you will understand immediately how nicotine causes changes to the reward system and makes you nicotine dependent.

Yet Smokers Continue to Believe Smoking Has Advantages

"Hmm, okay, so I smoke to occupy these receptors to feel normal again. But for a moment I definitely feel better than a nonsmoker." Precisely. You have hit the nail on the head. Instinctively, many smokers understand immediately how nicotine changes the reward center and how they systematically rid themselves of withdrawal symptoms by smoking. But in spite of this they are absolutely convinced that without nicotine they are denying themselves of something, of some "pleasure" they cannot obtain by any other means. That is why they cannot stop. Smokers are totally convinced that smoking has the advantages of having a calming effect in certain situations, lowering stress, increasing the power of concentration. They believe that for a short period of time, they not only reach the normal mood level of a nonsmoker, but exceed it. We will look at this paramount issue later: Does nicotine increase enjoyment or does it reduce your quality of life?

Nicotine During Pregnancy

The increased number of receptors can also be found in the children of mothers who smoked during pregnancy. The unborn child smokes along with the mother! It is no coincidence that the babies of mothers who smoke are often more restless and display more behavioral problems after birth compared to the babies of nonsmoking mothers. The former also show withdrawal symptoms.

Imagine how the brain cells of an unborn child grow, develop, divide, and multiply on a daily basis. The unbelievable miracle of life in creation and of developing cells is disturbed by nicotine. Nicotine can cause stimulation of neurotransmitters at the wrong times in brain development, which can stunt cell proliferation and cell growth. Animal experiments prove that certain areas of the brain have fewer nerve cells when nicotine is supplied.[23] In addition, the changes in the reward center of the brain, which you already know from your own nicotine

44

addiction, are more enduring in the developing brain. Children of mothers who smoke during pregnancy display more frequent behavioral problems and are more likely to have attention-deficit hyperactivity disorders (ADHD), and suffer more often from mood changes and depression.[24, 25, 26] Far too few women know how strongly smoking during pregnancy influences the mind and the reward system of the child, not only immediately after birth but for years to come.

THE BOTTOM LINE

- ▶ Nicotine occupies the receptors in the reward area of the brain. Excessive nicotine makes these insensitive and doubles the number of receptors.
- ▶ Due to this, the body is unable to produce enough transmitters to occupy all receptors and to stimulate the happiness transmitters sufficiently.
- ▶ For this reason, you must continue smoking just to feel normal, balanced, and satisfied—to get the feeling that you had for free before you started smoking.
- ▶ You smoke to rid yourself of restlessness and irritability, a deficiency of transmitters caused by nicotine, but you perceive this as a feeling of enjoyment, and as a reward.
- ▶ The lower the nicotine level, the more the smoker enjoys a subjective "improvement."

5

My Dog, My Children, My Wife . . .
The Uncomfortable Pressure of the Passive Smoker

My Dog . . .

It never really bothered me that someone else was passively smoking. And whenever I smoked, I thought, "If others find it annoying, then they don't have to stay beside me; they can move somewhere else. This whole thing about passive smoking is nothing but hysteria." Then I read in a newspaper article that dogs that are passive smokers are particularly at risk of getting cancer. Their exposure to smoke increases their risk of developing lung or nasal cancer by 60%. That made me think. My fox terrier, Robby, could not simply get up and leave the apartment as I sat puffing away in front of the television. I wasn't particularly worried about the fact I was endangering myself—okay, I did worry a bit—but that I was harming my dog did not please me at all. After reading that, I tried to confine my smoking to when I took Robby out for a walk around the block or to smoking only on the balcony.

According to a survey of over 3,000 households, one third of smokers said that the risk of their pet getting cancer would be a reason to quit smoking.[27] 1 in 4 nonsmokers would send their partner outside to smoke to make sure their pet was not put at risk. Yet for other nonsmokers, including their children, smokers showed little sympathy. In fact, in more than half the children living in homes where someone smokes, degradation products of nicotine could be detected in their urine. In a quarter of these cases, the amounts detected were equal to those found in barkeepers.[28]

Of course, I continued to smoke in the pub. Then came the smoking ban with all that nonsense about passive smoking. So, I was left standing outside on the sidewalk, freezing, where I dragged away on my cigarette feeling really pissed off. I really did not enjoy it at all. At least now and again, other smokers joined me in front of the door. "Smokers are more likeable anyway," I said to myself. "The spoilsports can keep to themselves. If only they could show just a little more tolerance." Many smokers get so fed up with dealing with smoking bans that it is a strong motivation for them to quit.

More Tolerance Required—The Lobby from the Tobacco Industry

Is passive smoking really so damaging to health? Is the time coming when smokers will practically not be allowed to smoke anywhere? For 15 years, the tobacco industry has been trying to play down the consequences of passive smoking as much as possible, making a joke of it, portraying nonsmokers as spoilsports. Expensive campaigns by the cigarette industry in Germany, such as "For More Tolerance" and "People, Culture, Pub," try time and again to boil the whole issue down to a simple lack of tolerance. That's logical. The biggest threat to tobacco industry profits is smoking bans on account of the risks of passive smoking. Studies commissioned by the tobacco industry tried to play down the risks of passive smoking. And not only were reputable German scientists bribed by the industry. So was the former head of the Federal Health Office in Berlin, Prof. Karl Überla. The studies that were commissioned were designed to obscure the risks of smoking and passive smoking. This, together with the lobbying done in the parliamentary committees, was meant to hinder the legal banning of smoking. This lobby was nowhere more successful than in Germany. Using "buy-and-sell commissioned studies," the multibillion-dollar tobacco industry followed the same pattern for decades. These manipulations by the drug dealers would be a great plot for a movie. Yet smokers just love to believe this scientific fraud and continue to ruin their health.

The Effects of Passive Smoking on Smokers, Themselves

Smokers in particular inhale the toxic sidestream smoke of the glowing cigarette between puffs. Passive smoke is known to be the most damaging and common indoor poison, comparable to the now banned asbestos as a toxic substance. Tobacco smoke has been shown to contain 90 carcinogenic substances. For the most part, these are Class I carcinogenic substances of which even the smallest amounts can cause cancer. There is no bottom limit or level that could be considered safe. These toxins are gaseous, invisible, and odorless. Thus, they go unnoticed. Only a very small number of them are perceptible as uncomfortable smoke particles. These toxins enter the body through inhalation. "I have children but I open the windows and air out the fumes," is the argument that many smokers tell me. But research show that even ventilating rooms for lengthy periods only disposes of a small fragment of these gaseous toxic substances. So if you have children you will not eliminate much of the toxins by opening the windows.

Some three quarters of a cigarette burns away as this highly toxic sidestream when the cigarette is just smoldering in the ashtray or in your hand. The concentration of toxic substances in sidestream smoke is 30 to 100 times higher in nitrosamines than it is in the mainstream smoke that the smoker inhales when drawing on the cigarette. What is the reason for this? It basically works like a waste incinerator: The temperature is the decisive factor to eliminate at least a part of the toxins. Mainstream smoke burns away the toxic substances better at 950°C than does the sidestream smoke, which has only half the temperature, at about 500°C. The longer a cigarette smolders away in the ashtray, the more its toxic substances are released as the tobacco is not burned quickly and completely. That is why sidestream smoke is 4 times more toxic than mainstream smoke—and, in addition, extremely carcinogenic. So the issue is far from one of tolerance, as the tobacco industry would have us believe in its expensive advertising campaigns. In closed spaces, you passively inhale the sidestream smoke of everyone's cigarettes. In the case of 14 cigarettes, this amounts to the carcinogenic substances contained in an additional 2.6 cigarettes.[29] Looking at it from this perspective, smoking outside on the balcony is "healthier" also for yourself.

My House, My Car, My Wife, My Children . . .

You all know immediately when you enter the car or home of a smoker—it stinks. But more important than the smell are the toxic substances, which are deposited everywhere. Smokers' cars are real toxic waste dumps. High concentrations of cadmium, lead, and nitrosamine can be found in house dust, furniture, carpets, even on wallpaper.

Toddlers in particular ingest 20 to 30 times more of these substances than do adults because they are crawling around on the floor and are much more susceptible on account of their low body weight. To expose children to these poisons is tantamount to physical assault, because the babies and children have no choice but to inhale the smoke. In Germany alone, some 60 young babies a year die from sudden infant death syndrome because their parents smoke. The children of smokers are more prone to asthma, pneumonia, and bronchitis than are the children of nonsmokers. And because children imitate their parents, those from families in which someone smokes are twice as likely to become smokers. Surely there is scarcely a smoker who wants to see his or her child dragging on a cigarette, yet smokers force them to inhale on a daily basis at home and in the car.

But as we've seen, the story is even worse for unborn children exposed to cigarette smoke during the mother's pregnancy. No one is more motivated to quit smoking than pregnant women are. As so many pregnant women wish to quit, I have included an extra info section on smoking and pregnancy on the website, and in this book.

Playing Down the Whole Issue

"I don't have any children and anyway this whole thing is exaggerated." Would you say the same thing if we were talking about the number of traffic deaths every year? Let's see the figures and how they compare: In 2009, there were 4,100 fatalities on the roads in Germany, and in the same year, 3,300 Germans died as a consequence of passive smoking.[30] In the United States, there are around 35,000 deaths annually from premature heart attacks and other diseases caused by passive smoking. After 30 years of sabotaging research, even the tobacco industry recognizes the validity of these numbers. Whoever shares a home with a smoker has a 25% to 30% greater risk of lethal heart disease and strokes and a 20% to 30% greater risk of lung cancer. The danger of passive smoking is very impressive and well researched. To learn more, please Google "passive smoking" in Wikipedia. I could not summarize this better."

Increasing Pressure on the Passive Smoker

"So, you are one of the militant nonsmoking lobby." No, by no means. But the facts on passive smoking will affect you and how you feel in the future as a smoker. You will come under increasing pressure. The times of smoking everywhere without giving it a thought are over. Nonsmokers have reconquered their sovereignty of the air through their long persistence and their right to have clean air. Now you have to apologize constantly for smoking or ask whether it is permitted to smoke. Now you have to retreat outside to smoke and harvest the unpleasant looks when caught smoking. Although as teenagers we found it cool to smoke, this has changed today. Emitting toxic substances and being addicted are becoming increasingly socially unacceptable and are not regarded as cool in the slightest. This hostile social environment was one of the main reasons for me to quit cigarettes. There are simply too many places where it is forbidden to smoke, and the restlessness when the nicotine level drops is a far from pleasant feeling.

Only for Pet Owners

Back again to Rover and Kitty. Cats lick their fur a lot and it is on the fur that these carcinogenic substances are deposited. A frequent consequence is mouth and lymph node cancer. After 5 years in a household where smokers live, the risk to cats of getting lymph node cancer increases threefold.[31] The risk is even quadrupled when there are 2 smokers in the house. In dogs, mainly the risk of lung and nasal cancer increases. Dogs with a long nose are at double the risk for nasal cancer, as the carcinogenic substances remain in the long nasal passages.[32] In short-nosed dogs, the substances usually get into the lungs. Birds are also extremely sensitive. In earlier years, birds were taken down mines to detect unnoticed leaking gases. If they died in their cage, the mine was evacuated immediately.

THE BOTTOM LINE

- ► The risks of passive smoking are clearly documented. This will mean that smoking will be banned in more and more locations.
- ► Smokers will come under more and more pressure.
- ► Smoking is becoming less and less a sociable habit, just a lonely routine just to feel normal again.

★ **CONGRATULATIONS!** You have just earned your first star and have completed the first part of the book. Maybe you had to have a few breaks when you put the book aside for a couple of days. That is normal. There is a lot to digest. In spite of resistance, you have come this far. Bravo! You are on the right path.

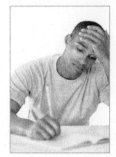

Part 2

Smoking

and the

Mind

6

The Daily Ups
and Downs
Caused by Nicotine

FOR MANY, THE FIRST CIGARETTE OF the day is
the best one. You get up still tired and in slightly dampened
spirits, make a coffee, smoke a cigarette as a jump starter, and
already you feel more awake; your overall spirits and mood
improve. You get into gear, thanks to that cigarette.

When do you start smoking each day? Immediately after you
get up, to get a better start? Always with a coffee? Or is it later in
the day? This tells a lot about how addicted your body has
become to nicotine. Take the short Fagerström Test.

Fagerström Test of Tobacco Dependency

How soon after you wake up do you smoke your first cigarette?

Within 5 minutes	❏ 3
Within 6 to 30 minutes	❏ 2
Within 31 to 60 minutes	❏ 1
After 60 minutes	❏ 0

Do you find it difficult to refrain from smoking in places where it is prohibited (e.g., cinemas, pubs, trains)?

Yes	❏ 1
No	❏ 0

Which cigarette would you hate to give up?

The first one in the morning	❏ 1
Others	❏ 0

Generally, how many cigarettes do you smoke daily?

Up to 10	❏ 0
11 to 20	❏ 1
21 to 30	❏ 2
31 or more	❏ 3

Do you smoke more frequently in the first hours after getting up than during the rest of the day?

Yes	❏ 1
No	❏ 0

Do you smoke when you have a cold or are ill and have to stay in bed all day?

Yes	❏ 1
No	❏ 0

Total points   _____

Evaluation of the Fagerström Test of Tobacco Dependency

This test shows your degree of dependency. But it cannot say whether your chances are better or worse to succeed at quitting smoking. A light smoker with little psychological strain may find quitting much more difficult than might a heavy smoker who hates the monotony of having to smoke. The more addicted you are, the more restless, irritable, nervous, and in certain cases, less energetic and less concentrated you feel, even in the shortest periods of nicotine withdrawal.

People revert to smoking cigarettes

- to reduce stress
- to improve mood and the feeling of well-being
- to have more energy to get through the day
- to concentrate better

Because these are the 4 most commonly stated reasons to smoke, I've made them the topics of this chapter.

How Many Points Did You Score?

0–2 POINTS—LOW DEPENDENCY: You have conditioned yourself to smoke in certain situations; for example, after eating or in the company of friends. Your physical dependency is low. You do not feel pressured to smoke a cigarette first thing in the morning. Sometimes you go without a cigarette until the afternoon, evening, or the following day. You don't have mood swings due to low nicotine levels and don't smoke to control these addiction mood swings. You rarely use cigarettes to cope with stress and don't need nicotine as a jump start to be able to concentrate. In spite of this, you find it difficult to quit smoking. Only 15% to 20% of smokers belong to the group of light smokers, although many smokers see themselves as belonging to this group. Few light smokers remain at this level of smoking for a long time. Some force themselves to smoke at this low level.

3–5 POINTS—MEDIUM DEPENDENCY: You smoke for "enjoyment" and sometimes more often in stressful situations. Some medium-dependency smokers start to control their mood swings more and more often with nicotine. Others, but not all, already smoke in the morning for stimulation, or later in the day to be able to concentrate better.

6–7 POINTS—HIGH DEPENDENCY: You often smoke cigarettes to improve your mood or sense of well-being, "to give yourself a treat," and in stressful situations. Cigarettes help many high-dependency smokers to get through the day when they are tired or want to concentrate. Nicotine improves their mood in the morning and some can only get started with nicotine.

8–10 POINTS—VERY HIGH DEPENDENCY: You cannot imagine life without smoking. You smoke first thing in the morning to get the day started and to overcome tiredness. You quickly get into a bad mood if you cannot smoke. You have trouble coping with stress without the help of a cigarette. When you know that you will not be able to smoke for a longer period of time, you top up your nicotine reserves beforehand. An empty pack in the evening can cause restlessness, fear, or even panic.

The Fortune and Misfortune of the Light Smoker

Are you a light smoker? Then you are both lucky and unlucky. Your physical dependence is low. You don't experience an emotional roller coaster when you don't smoke, but may feel very little pressure to really quit smoking. Chances are, however, that you don't want to do without a cigarette after a meal or when in the company of friends. In chapter 11, I will show you how nicotine addiction has managed to anchor itself as a strong desire to smoke in certain situations. If you really want to quit smoking, you must consciously train yourself to get rid of the conditioned cues that make you smoke.

Medium to More Dependent Smokers

Most smokers, despite perhaps viewing themselves as light smokers, actually fall into the group of medium to more dependent smokers. One obvious clue: Why does the first cigarette in the morning feel so good? The answer is simple: In the morning, you have the greatest nicotine deficit. Due to this, you may not want to do without your first cigarette. Otherwise, the day is off to a bad start. This need signals your physical dependency.

The Slight Feeling of Emptiness

80% of smokers agree with the following statements:[33] "Smoking relaxes me"; "Smoking has a calming effect"; "I do not feel content if I haven't smoked for a while." Well-being, feeling better, and mood control are important reasons for smoking. Why? After even a short period of time, a lower nicotine level in the blood causes a slight feeling of restlessness. Something seems to be missing. Your mood deteriorates. This feeling can be so unnoticeable that you are scarcely conscious of it; it intensifies until you want to "enjoy" the next cigarette. Depending on how dependent you are, you will feel fairly stressed, nervous, on edge, and even unconcentrated after just 30 minutes of not smoking. The desire to smoke a cigarette *now*, to get rid of these feelings, continues to increase.

Over the years, after smoking thousands of cigarettes, you have learned to avoid these minimal feelings of restlessness. You have learned to top up automatically with nicotine. The relaxation and enjoyment comes primarily from having this feeling of restlessness disappear. This does not mean that you feel better in comparison to nonsmokers. But you do feel better compared to the tension that built up before you smoked.

Let´s further look at this situation: Does smoking just relieve your withdrawal symptoms temporarily? Or is the cigarette a real gain, enhancing mood and concentration? Most smokers concede that cigarettes are unhealthy but are convinced that cigarette are an indispensable and unique source of enjoyment and a real gain to their sense of well-being. This is why no smoker wants to do without them. For smokers, there is nothing better than a good cigarette. We are really all about our cigarettes.

The Daily Ups and Downs

Let's take a look at a smoker's day. You already know: The degree of enjoyment depends directly on your nicotine level. At the beginning of the 80s, systematic research was done into the "experienced desire" to smoke. With the first cigarette in the morning, you first fill the nicotine gap. With deep and long inhalations you try to counterbalance the reduction of your nicotine level of the previous night. Maximum enjoyment.

And what about cigarettes after that? How is each following cigarette evaluated—not like the 6-hour smoking test on page 30 under laboratory conditions, but on a day when you can smoke as many as you want?

Prof. Andrew C. Parrott made a study of the relationship of smoking and stress. 105 smokers gave their evaluation, based on a scale assessing tension and nervousness before and after a cigarette.[34] The assessment scale was as follows: 2-1-0-1-2 from *tense* to *relaxed* and 2-1-0-1-2 from *nervous* to *calm*. After each cigarette, the medium to heavy smoker felt less tense and less nervous than before smoking a cigarette. We all know that feeling: After a cigarette, we feel an improvement and interpret this as enjoyment, which is stored in the brain as a short-term benefit. But what are we really looking at? We can see that smokers are constantly fluctuating between *tense/nervous* before a cigarette and *relaxed/*

calm after a cigarette. It's a constant up and down. This was felt throughout every day with every single cigarette by the 105 smokers and the study assessed this precisely.

The regularity of these falling curves in the case of every single smoker surprised Prof. Parrott. This constant up and down of tension causes enormous additional stress in smokers at the end of the day, a form of stress that nonsmokers just do not experience. So it was no surprise that when several thousand additional smokers were questioned, almost half of them, 47%, stated they smoked to reduce stress.[35] Yes, stress is *caused* by smoking and the shortsighted solution is to relieve this by additional smoking!

Not a Plateau but an Increased Up and Down

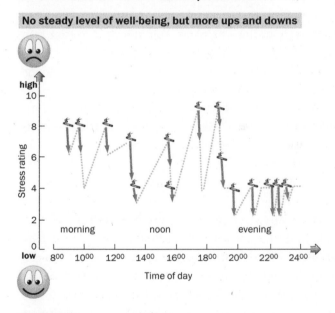

No steady level of well-being, but more ups and downs

🔥 Cigarette

⋯⋯ Abstinence between cigarettes

A constant up and down. Here you can see a typical stress progression of someone who participated in the study: tension/nervousness before smoking ➞ relaxation/calmness afterward ➞ renewed increase between cigarettes, spread over the study participant's day.

Not a Plateau but an Increased Up and Down

The study also shows that you don't smoke to attain a longer-lasting, satisfied feeling and then decide voluntarily when to light up the next cigarette. The story is entirely different: The increasing tension prior to each cigarette produces the desire for another cigarette. The longer you wait, the greater the desire becomes, the greater the compulsion to smoke another cigarette . . . to smoke a cigarette *now*. Your enjoyment/relaxation is mainly relief from the prior tension. This demonstrates the enormous psychological dependency caused by nicotine.

At the time of the greatest nicotine deficit, after a night without cigarettes, mood is improved most rapidly with the first cigarette in the morning. But smokers experience other ups and downs throughout the whole day. You know the reason from reading the previous chapter: the receptors in the brain, which have become desensitized and changed by nicotine, are no longer sufficiently stimulated without nicotine. The result is a lack of happiness transmitters. Without nicotine, you have a chronic feeling of dissatisfaction. This shift in the reward center of the brain makes you reach for the next cigarette.

Between Feeling Tired and Stimulated

Apart from tension and relaxation, many but not all smokers feel stimulated and have more drive after smoking: "I just get through my day better"; "Otherwise I can't get myself into gear in the morning"; "I can simply concentrate better"; "I always smoke when I feel tired." In the study with the 105 smokers, especially with the heavy smokers, a precise smoking pattern is even more frequently visible. Smokers who feel somewhat tired *before* smoking are more awake and have more energy *after* a cigarette. But another issue that emerged is much more interesting: *Between* cigarettes, the feeling of stimulation decreases very quickly. This creates a much stronger up and down of the energy and concentration levels in smokers, in comparison to nonsmokers. The constant fluctuation from feeling down to feeling better after having smoked a cigarette, and the subsequent return to the original state of feeling down, turns a smoker's day into a stamina competition. That causes stress—big time!

Stress and Boredom

"I smoke when I am stressed, but also when I am alone or bored." Smoking causes a double stress: especially in already stressful situations, additional stress is felt most acutely when there is a low level of nicotine in the body. You want to smoke to relieve this additional stress as quickly as possible.

But even perfectly calm situations can give rise to the desire for a cigarette. Particularly when you are not distracted, the restlessness and tension caused by a low level of nicotine is felt more quickly: "I overcome boredom with a cigarette." Yes, smoking is an activity. But just how interesting is this automated activity, really? Boredom is a psychological state that is not much alleviated by smoking. You might as well listen to music, watch TV, play with your smart phone, or do something else, without lighting up. These activities don't become more interesting or less boring because you just happen to be holding a cigarette between your fingers.

"And what if I do nothing and just want to think things over?"; "Cigarettes relax me when I have moments of leisure." What's really happening is that without distraction, you are more aware of your withdrawal symptoms and want to get rid of these as quickly as possible so as to relax again or think more calmly.

The Winning Theory: Enjoyment or Loss

"Okay. Smokers have mood swings and ups and downs in tension and energy, but when all is said and done, these improve after each cigarette. That is exactly why I enjoy smoking and would miss it." So do smokers really feel better than nonsmokers? At the end of the day, do smokers experience more enjoyment and have a better mood than nonsmokers? Are they more relaxed? Do they have less stress? This has been investigated using various models:

THE WINNING MODEL: Some smokers are convinced that smoking has benefits in terms of enjoyment, well-being, relaxation, and concentration. With every cigarette they smoke, smokers would rise above the line showing the mean value.

This line shows how nonsmokers rate their state of mind. Convinced smokers believe that perhaps their mood, sense of feeling relaxed, and powers of concentration drop somewhat between cigarettes, but that overall they have an advantage over nonsmokers.

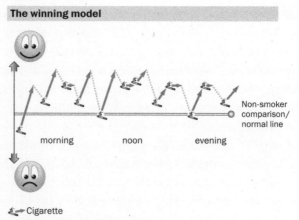

The winning model

morning   noon   evening

Non-smoker comparison/ normal line

🚬 Cigarette

······ Abstinence between cigarettes

The "I enjoy smoking" model

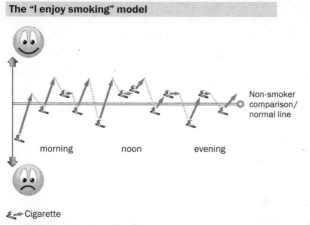

morning   noon   evening

Non-smoker comparison/ normal line

🚬← Cigarette

······ Abstinence between cigarettes

THE "I ENJOY SMOKING" MODEL: The second chart matches the convictions of most smokers: "I feel better than a nonsmoker [black line], but especially when I feel worse, I have cigarettes as a support. They make me more relaxed, make me feel better, can alleviate stress quickly, and I enjoy the present moment more. In these moments of enjoyment I definitely feel better than nonsmokers. So I would constantly miss cigarettes if I were to quit."

THE AVOIDANCE/WITHDRAWAL MODEL: Even after a short period without a cigarette, smokers feel more nervous, uneasy, grumpy, more stressed, less energetic, and less concentrated or focused. They have learned to alleviate these mild withdrawal symptoms through smoking in order to feel relaxed again. At best, smokers can reach the same normal levels of nonsmokers. The stronger the dependence and the longer they have been smoking, the stronger this avoidance is. It's been learned through millions of puffs on a cigarette. This blends into an automatic smoking behavior.

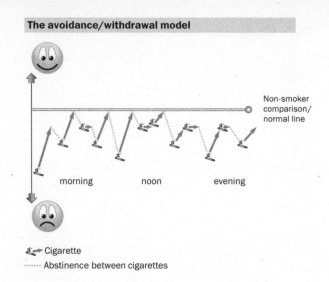

The avoidance/withdrawal model

Non-smoker
comparison/
normal line

morning   noon   evening

Cigarette
...... Abstinence between cigarettes

The Winning and the "I Enjoy Smoking" Models

In what category would you place yourself? The "I enjoy smoking" model corresponds to the satisfaction and subjective experience of most smokers. But let's think one step further: If the psychological benefits of smoking, in which I also believed, are really true, then certain assumptions must automatically be true:

- If a smoking benefit does exist, then smokers must feel less stressed, have a generally better state of mind, and have an overall higher joie de vivre than nonsmokers.
- Through improved concentration after a cigarette, smokers would have to perform better intellectually than nonsmokers.
- If smoking is an asset, one should be able to identify more enjoyment and a better or at least equally

balanced mood and less stress among young people after they've started smoking.

- But, most important of all, if smoking has benefits, then smokers who have quit must feel less satisfied than they previously did, and experience less enjoyment and pleasure and more stress and a general poorer state of mind.

These assumptions have been systematically researched over the last 30 years. To do so, both smokers and nonsmokers were interviewed and their responses compared:

- 3 groups were compared: smokers experiencing mild withdrawal symptoms, smokers who just had a cigarette, and nonsmokers.
- The mood and stress levels of young people were compared before they started smoking and after they had become smokers.
- The stress levels, mood, and satisfaction of smokers who quit were monitored and these were compared "before quitting" and "several weeks after quitting."

You Cannot Compare Apples to Oranges

The issue is not whether the *psychological* advantages of smoking outweigh the *physical* damage it causes. That would be comparing apples to oranges and would be a useless exercise for smokers. Every "smoker inquisition" by a nonsmoker begins with this apples and oranges comparison; in other words, the dangers of smoking to health. Health is one important reason for quitting. It provides major motivation. But nothing more than that. Still it fails to answer the question of why we enjoy smoking so much. In my seminars, smokers are much more interested in asking whether they have to forgo this psychological benefit/enjoyment they have acquired: "If I want to relax I'll miss smoking . . ."; "When I want to feel better or am in a bad mood, I enjoy a cigarette"; "When I want to treat myself . . . I will miss being able to have a cigarette"; "I've always liked smoking and have been satisfied by a cigarette—if I quit smoking . . . will I always have the feeling of missing out on something?"; "Stress without a cigarette . . . I don't know if I could manage . . . "; "How can I get through the day without a cigarette?"; "When I feel lousy and can't concentrate I like smoking . . . what should I do instead?"

Every smoker knows the feeling of these advantages and the enjoyment from smoking a cigarette. But are they really advantages? Does nicotine make you feel more satisfied, less stressed? Does it increase your concentration and ability to perform compared to nonsmokers without nicotine? Do you get above the normal line or remain below it? We will learn more about this in the following chapter.

THE BOTTOM LINE

- ▶ The stronger the nicotine addiction, the more prone the smoker is to stress and to severe mood, energy, and concentration fluctuations. Nicotine is used to stop these nervous fluctuations.
- ▶ Smokers perceive to have "benefits" after smoking a cigarette, but don´t think about the reduction of these said "benefits" between cigarettes.
- ▶ The falling level of nicotine in the body increases restlessness, pressure, and stress until the dulled docking areas in the brain absorb more nicotine.
- ▶ Throughout the day, smokers experience constant ups and downs, with tension and restlessness.

7

Smoking with No Advantages

Relaxation, Stress Reduction, and Improvement of Mood

"Well, I enjoy smoking. Quitting smoking would be a loss for me. You can't convince me that I've been wrong for 20 years, and that by smoking I only reach the same baseline level of satisfaction as a nonsmoker. You'll have to prove that before I'll believe it."

Give me just 10 minutes of your time and I will.

The Psychobiological Effect of Nicotine

The key issue: If you smoke, do you feel better than a nonsmoker in absolute terms? Prof. Parrott has researched this matter. He is one of the pioneers in researching the psychobiological effects of nicotine in smokers. In his experiments, 3 groups assessed their state of mind:

1. Smokers who continue to smoke normally without nicotine withdrawal
2. Smokers after 12 hours of nicotine withdrawal
3. nonsmokers

This assessment happened *before* a performance test and *after* a 10-minute pause.[36] This questionnaire on the 3 most important mood factors for smokers—stress, well-being, and stimulation—has proven to be a reliable and significant tool over many years. Stay with me—this will really catch your interest!

STRESS: **TENSE**	❑ very	❑ somewhat	❑ neither	❑ somewhat	❑ very **RELAXED**
NERVOUS:	❑ very	❑ somewhat	❑ neither	❑ somewhat	❑ very **CALM**
STIMULATION: **ENERGETIC**	❑ very	❑ somewhat	❑ neither	❑ somewhat	❑ very **TIRED**
ALERT:	❑ very	❑ somewhat	❑ neither	❑ somewhat	❑ very **DROWSY**
PLEASURE: **SATISFIED**	❑ very	❑ somewhat	❑ neither	❑ somewhat	❑ very **DISSATISFIED**
CONTENT:	❑ very	❑ somewhat	❑ neither	❑ somewhat	❑ very **IRRITATED**

This Is How Smokers Really Assess Their Mood?

The initial assessment of the mood scale in the study shows that smokers who have not smoked for a longer period are more tense, more nervous, less satisfied, and less content than non-smokers or smokers without nicotine withdrawal. That is obvious. You know that yourself: The longer you haven't smoked, the grumpier you become. In contrast to this, nonsmokers as well as smokers who smoke normally share identical results in the mood test. Smokers with high levels of nicotine do not rank the 3 areas of stress, stimulation, and well-being any better than do nonsmokers in the 3 areas of stress, stimulation, and well-being.

This shows that nicotine provides no benefits to them, compared to the mood results of nonsmokers.

This mood assessment was followed by a short performance test and then a second mood assessment after a break for a cigarette. The second cigarette produced no extra benefit to smokers who have no nicotine withdrawal, as compared to nonsmokers, in the mood areas of stress, stimulation, and well-being. The second assessment shows no improvement in these smokers, as the short interval between both cigarettes was not long enough to produce a markedly falling nicotine level and accompanying withdrawal symptoms. In contrast, the smokers with overnight nicotine withdrawal showed significant improvement in all 3 mood areas. They have now at last reached the normal level of nonsmokers and smokers who have no nicotine deficit. Take a look at this again in the graph. ("Oh no, not another graph.") Really, it's interesting and much easier to comprehend if you take a look. Here, nicotine produces no increase above the normal level of mood. That nicotine improves mood is—and remains—purely an assumption on the part of smokers, not borne out by the assessment results. All nicotine does is relieve you of the unpleasant feelings of withdrawal.

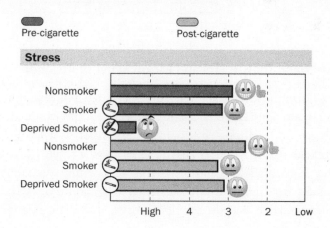

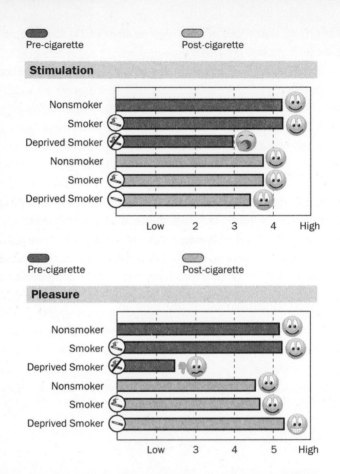

Summary: Only a Normal Mood Level Is Attained

If the nicotine level is low, smokers only reach a normal mood level by smoking and then feel just as relaxed, calm, stimulated, satisfied, and comfortable as nonsmokers. Smokers who smoke to relieve strong withdrawal symptoms show a slightly higher value for "satisfied" than do smokers who continue to smoke while having a high nicotine base level for a short time. That is understandable, because the relief provided by the cigarette is greater. In the pleasure graph, we see quite clearly that nicotine intake does nothing more than restore normal levels and that smokers have no advantage over nonsmokers in terms of stress, stimulation, or pleasure. The benefit to the smoker is nothing more than a subjective "felt benefit" the more he or she smokes to get rid of withdrawal symptoms.

What Does Smoking Improve?

The study examined not only mood but also the withdrawal symptoms most frequently mentioned by smokers when they cannot smoke. It is these very withdrawal symptoms that push us to continue smoking. Again, (1) smokers without nicotine withdrawal symptoms, (2) smokers with nicotine withdrawal symptoms before and after the cigarette break, and (3) nonsmokers assess these withdrawal symptoms.

RESTLESSNESS:	❏ extremely	❏ very	❏ somewhat	❏ slightly	❏ not at all
BAD MOOD/ DEPRESSION:	❏ extremely	❏ very	❏ somewhat	❏ slightly	❏ not at all
IRRITABILITY:	❏ extremely	❏ very	❏ somewhat	❏ slightly	❏ not at all
POOR CONCENTRATION:	❏ extremely	❏ very	❏ somewhat	❏ slightly	❏ not at all
HUNGER:	❏ extremely	❏ very	❏ somewhat	❏ slightly	❏ not at all
URGE TO SMOKE:	❏ extremely	❏ very	❏ somewhat	❏ slightly	❏ not at all

Again, there is no difference between smokers (with no nicotine deprivation) and nonsmokers. As long as there is enough nicotine in their blood, smokers are not more restless, in a worse mood, more irritable, or less concentrated. Both groups rate their moods similarly. This explains why smokers are socially acceptable in contrast to those taking most other addictive drugs. Smokers are and feel completely normal as long as they are on nicotine. They remain capable of working. On the other hand . . . what an unoriginal drug, when you're paying a fortune for nicotine only to reach a normal state of mind.

In contrast to this, smokers experiencing nicotine withdrawal before the cigarette are more restless, have a worse mood, are more irritable, and have less ability to concentrate. Only after smoking a cigarette does this restlessness, bad mood, poor concentration, and irritability decrease to levels that are regular for nonsmokers.

Smoking to Stop Withdrawal Symptoms

Please, take another look at the bar graphs for smokers that are suffering withdrawal. After one whole night without smoking, the nicotine level could not be completely compensated for by a single cigarette. Smokers with severe withdrawal symptoms also differ from the group that smokes regularly: They are always in a worse mood and more irritable than the other smokers. These smokers feel this quite clearly. For this reason, they assess the withdrawal symptom "urge to smoke" significantly higher than do the smokers who have already smoked on that day. This unremitting desire for a cigarette is the precise feeling for the need to continue smoking to rid oneself of the bad feeling, the withdrawal symptoms. The nicotine after the first cigarette has not sufficiently stabilized their normal level of well-being. I am certain you are aware of this in yourself when you have to refuel with nicotine after a long flight. Or, conversely, the "avoidance strategy": smoking several cigarettes before a flight to keep the nicotine level as high as possible, so that you suffer less later. But, in all honesty, this has little to do with enjoyment and pleasure.

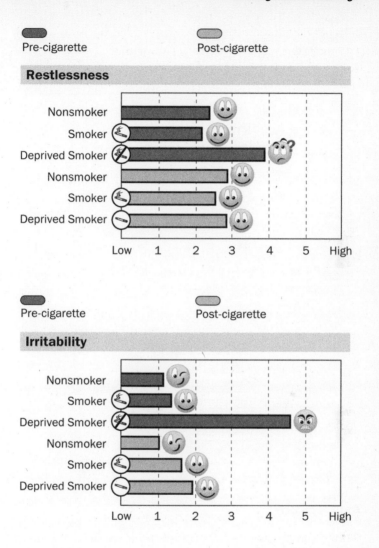

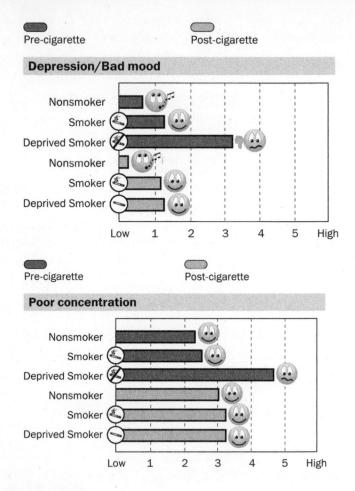

Too Detailed?

"Hmm, couldn't you say all that with fewer words?" Of course I could, but you would have to "believe" the sentence, "Instead of getting pleasure from smoking, you are only relieving your withdrawal symptoms." But that would only work with your having good faith in that statement. Most smokers are firmly convinced of the pleasure and benefits of smoking. Quickly, the addicted brain pipes up and does everything to continue to convince you that such a sentence is false. I don't want you to "believe" any-thing I say. We are not in church. The mechanisms of drug addiction have been well researched. These graphs show exactly how nicotine plays with your emotions and that you just reach a normal level of well-being that you had for free before you started smoking.

Summary: The Vicious Cycle of Mood Swings

The relaxing and stress-reducing effect of smoking consists only of normalizing withdrawal symptoms, such as restlessness and irritability. Smoking is also satisfying because it improves a bad mood, which is a withdrawal symptom. The smoker smokes to attain a normal feeling of well-being equal to that of a nonsmoker. But smokers were not calmer, did not have better moods, and were no less irritable than nonsmokers. In actual fact, smokers are prone to a much stronger, constant up and down of mood swings, which they try to overcome by continu-ing to smoke.

In the performance tests that were given during the central portion of Parrott's study, smokers did not have better powers of concentration than did nonsmokers who had this for free with-out the aid of cigarettes.

Throughout the Day: Stress, Stimulation, and Enjoyment

"Regardless—I am sure that I still get through the day better with cigarettes. They are a real help. This study assessed only one small part of the day. Perhaps in looking at the whole course of the day, smokers feel better than nonsmokers." This is another interesting question and has been researched on sev-eral occasions by comparing the mood levels of smokers and nonsmokers every 2 to 3 hours throughout the day. The best results obtained in one of these studies showed that smokers who were allowed to smoke and nonsmokers did not differ in the levels of stress, stimulation, or pleasure when being assessed every 3 hours.[37]

On the other hand, many other studies prove that, depending on the degree of dependency of the smoker (assessed every 2 hours), the assessed mood is worse. This is due to the constant mood fluctuations. In addition, in these studies, heavy smokers rated their state of mind worse than did those who smoked a moderate number of cigarettes. Nonsmokers constantly rated their mood better.[38]

When all is said and done: By smoking you can at best attain a normal level of well-being. Many achieve lower than this, particularly those who are heavily dependent. In addition, they go through the day with more severe mood fluctuations than nonsmokers.

Smoking More on Stressful Days

"Okay, but all these are laboratory studies. I would like to see what the situation is in everyday life." You are right. The daily "little annoyances and hassles" cause the most stress. Stress at work, stress with colleagues, quarrels in the family always about the same thing, relationship problems that cannot seem to be resolved, long travel times to work—we are all caught up daily in constant mini-stress situations that wear us down, make us grumpy, and give us a bad mood. However, smokers who are stressed tend to reach for a cigarette to overcome a bad mood and relieve stress. To relax. Smoking seems like a stress valve, a benefit, and it does help—temporarily. When under stress, smokers inhale more rapidly and more deeply to attain the desired effect. The rapid influx of nicotine has an initially relaxing effect. But only for a short time! In thousands of situations you have learned and stored this in your brain:

severe stress ⟶ *mood deterioration and stimulation* ⟶ *need to smoke* ⟶ *short-lived relaxation.* Smoking does not relieve the causes of your stress, which will remain once the nicotine in your body ebbs.

Ask Smokers in Real Life

Does mood really improve by smoking when stressed? Here you have to ask smokers in real life: smokers who have fought with the daily little annoyances—a stressful life perhaps comparable to your own—and wanted to feel better by smoking a cigarette. In one sophisticated study of this issue, 256 smokers were interviewed in depth by telephone on 8 consecutive days. That made for a total of 2,048 interviews with targeted questions about daily stress (frequency, duration), how the smokers personally assessed their stress and their mood fluctuations (I feel tense, I couldn't care less, I feel nervous/restless/sad/overexerted, nothing could cheer me up, etc.), as well as smoking behavior (when and how many). What was the result?

You already know: Smokers smoke to avoid the slightest feeling of nervous withdrawal symptoms. When the nicotine deficit has been eliminated, additional cigarettes do not cause any improvement in mood.[39]

When confronted with too severe everyday stress, we are more prone to possible mood fluctuations and nervousness, due to withdrawal symptoms. What is the simplest solution? We continue smoking to avoid the symptoms. One problem less to deal with. Both—stress and restlessness caused by a fluctuating nicotine level—would simply be too much to deal with. We have to feel at our best now. High nicotine level + relaxing effect = better mood. But that is precisely wrong.

By means of the 2,048 in-depth telephone interviews, the relationship between smoking and stress on days that had a similar high stress level could be evaluated. Notably, the participants could not always smoke the same number of cigarettes on high-stress days. Perhaps they didn't manage to have a cigarette outside or were unable to take a smoking break. And precisely this difference is interesting in regard to the question of whether smoking more causes a greater reduction in stress. The result was amazing: When smokers smoked more than usual on days when they encountered stress, they were likely to feel emotionally worse off. Why? Smoking in itself causes stress. It increases the heart rate and blood pressure. Release of adrenaline and the stress hormone cortisol also increases. On stressful days, this additional stress from smoking, itself, has a significant effect on moods. As the study showed, we feel a temporary improvement in mood lasting from 10 to 15 minutes, but when everything is taken into consideration for the entire day, the mood caused by smoking stress is always worse.

Summary: Smoking Increases Stress

It is simply an illusion to believe that nicotine provides us with support in severe stress situations. The opposite is true:

Severe stress + withdrawal stress →

deterioration in mood + added tension →

the desire to smoke →

an increase in smoking to completely eliminate the withdrawal stress →

a short period of relaxation but increased physiological stress due to nicotine's side effects →

an overall high level of stress and deterioration in mood.

Smoking Always Causes Stress, Even If You Are Not Directly Aware of It

"But, if this were true, then on days where I have little stress and smoke a lot, my mood should deteriorate." How you perceive additional stress depends overall on your condition on the day and the overall stress. On some days, even the traffic in front of your office gets on your nerves, and on other days, you don't even hear it. The same holds true for smoking stress caused by too many cigarettes: you can cope with it better on good days than on others. And I do mean "cope with." At some point, the decreasing amount of oxygen suppressed by the carbon dioxide will take its toll, apart from that smoking steadily increases your levels of adrenaline and cortisol. Your constantly increasing heart rate will be perceived, at least subconsciously, as stress.

THE HB MAN—A SMOKER IN WITHDRAWAL

HB is a famous German cigarette brand. A long-running TV campaign was a comic strip in which the leading character—the HB man—always got completely worked up under stress, almost had a nervous breakdown, and then smoked a cigarette to come down again. Have a look at these advertisements on the Internet program. The HB man is the prototype for nervous, irritable withdrawal symptoms. Between the initial stress of his situation and the stress of withdrawal, he's put doubly under pressure, until eventually he explodes again. That's the vicious circle of falling nicotine levels. There are no psychological benefits to nicotine: The more you are addicted, the more it affects your mood and the more often you become overburdened, nervous, and ill-tempered. Don't miss these ads.

Smoking Makes You Feel Smaller

"If it makes us more irritable, why do so many people still reach for a cigarette?" On 1 pack a day, your brain learns, in the course of 70,000 or 80,000 puffs every year, how it can waft away tension, unrest, and discontent in only a few seconds, while satisfaction and well-being increase. Unconsciously, you will always reach for that pack.

> How many cigarettes have you actually consciously smoked today? _____
>
> And how many are missing from the box and were smoked on autopilot? _____

The greater the withdrawal, the greater the perceived release of tension and the "enjoyment." Over the course of years of conditioning, feelings of withdrawal come to be felt as moods that may be avoided. By and by, these shifts in mood tend to be seen as resulting from your own disposition, your nervousness and susceptibility to stress written off as innate personality traits. In fact, it is cigarettes that lie at the root of these mood swings. After millions of puffs, once smoking has become second nature, you come to believe that the cigarettes can put an end to these mood swings and this tension, indeed that you must smoke so as to cope with them. After 20 or 30 years of smoking, you'll hardly be able to even remember how you could ever have been relaxed without a cigarette in your mouth. The cigarette becomes your paid assistant; you feel too weak or short on willpower to make it without smoking, let alone to quit completely. And herein lies the most humiliating blow for the smoker's psyche: It strikes at self-confidence and self-esteem, as the smokers ascribe their weakness to themselves. Many smokers are aware of the physical damage caused by smoking, but few are aware of its psychological toll. Smoking provides no benefits; it has a destructive effect on your psyche, on your daily well-being, your self-confidence, and self-esteem!

It is thus hardly a surprise that, after only a few weeks' abstention, smokers notice their tension, stress, and irritability decline, and feel more content and balanced. In addition, they experience feelings of pride, of self-confidence at having freed themselves from the slavery of nicotine. You, too, can enjoy this new freedom every day.

In chapter 9, I will show you how smokers in research studies noticed exactly this improvement upon quitting. After all, this isn't about believing me, but about knowing the facts.

> *What one has learned to understand, one no longer fears.*
> —Marie Curie

The Electronic Cigarette

With the assistance of Hollywood, tobacco producers are trying to make a new addictive product fashionable: The electronic cigarette nebulizes a nicotine capsule with tobacco scent, but produces no bothersome smoke. The highest-paid movie stars in the world demonstrate this product to gullible consumers: In the middle of the film *The Tourist*, Johnny Depp explains at length to Angelina Jolie how the electronic cigarette works, and contentedly puffs away his addiction. After this chapter, I think it should be clear that nicotine has *no* benefits for your psyche, and that the electronic cigarette simply draws out the daily withdrawal struggle and the roller coaster of mood swings. You need an electronic cigarette as little as you need any other kind.

The Symptoms of Addiction

What is one of the main characteristics of all addictive drugs? After a certain time, users take the drugs mainly to avoid the unpleasant symptoms of withdrawal. The junkie is soon shooting up not for a high, but to avoid the excruciating pain of withdrawal. For heroin users, withdrawal is such a terrible experience that others clearly notice it.

Unlike heroin, nicotine doesn't cause much of a "high" in new users. Smoking is a social phenomenon: Smokers take it up to seem cool and grown-up, to rebel, to belong—and, at first, it takes practice. How is a smoker supposed to describe the effects of cigarettes if there's no high? How to explain the overwhelming yearning for a cigarette if, after smoking, one merely feels normal? In this way, the effect of nicotine is usually described simply as "enjoyment" and "satisfying," even if it's only a return to normal. This is also why a nonsmoker, whose brain has not been reprogrammed by addiction, cannot understand cigarettes' appeal. Just as with all other drugs, this "enjoyment" repeated on an hourly basis is primarily about the avoidance of the sensations associated with withdrawal, which you only experience if hooked in the first place.

Smoking and the Need to Refuel

The need to keep up supply is just the same as it is with other drugs. The old advertising slogan, "I'd walk a mile for a Camel," describes nothing more than the need to keep a supply of drugs on hand to avoid feelings of withdrawal. Have you never walked in the pouring rain to the store or driven to the gas station late at night to buy cigarettes? In such situations, I've even tried to relight stubbed-out butts from the ashtray, or bummed a cigarette from complete strangers. We rarely wish to sink so low. We try to avoid these feelings of withdrawal at almost any cost, by always having cigarettes close at hand, hoarding them in our pockets and storing them at home. And the cigarette industry takes pity on smokers in need: Its 800,000 machines give Germany the densest network of cigarette vending machines in Europe. And every smoker is "understanding," usually "helping out" and sharing a smoke with a stranger. But, only for the "enjoyment," of course. This false conception of "enjoyment" goes so far that, until 2010, cigarettes were counted as part of the basket of goods used to calculate welfare payments for the long-term unemployed in Germany.

THE BOTTOM LINE

- ▶ With low levels of nicotine in their blood, smokers are below the normal line of well-being, as compared with nonsmokers.
- ▶ The perceived feeling of improvement after inhaling nicotine gets the smoker up to the same balanced level as a nonsmoker, but no higher.
- ▶ Nicotine has no beneficial effect on the psyche, but causes sharp swings in satisfaction levels.
- ▶ The enjoyment, relaxation, stress relief, and inspiration or stimulation allegedly caused by smoking cigarettes are nothing else than a temporary relief from withdrawal symptoms.
- ▶ Cigarettes don't reduce stress; rather, they increase it.
- ▶ After a few years, smokers blame their mood shifts and susceptibility to stress on their own personality, rather than accepting nicotine addiction as the cause of these fluctuations.

The Stimulation and Concentration Myth

HAVE YOU PERHAPS GOT A NONSMOKING partner and been caught up in a conversation first thing in the morning, when all you want to do is start the day with a quiet cigarette? Have you ever gone on vacation with nonsmoking friends and been irritated by their degree of energy in the mornings, when you just wanted to have your morning smoke? Tolerant smokers overlook these excessively chipper morning people, and, in time, come to think that they simply aren't a morning person with energy and mental activity to spare early in the day. But is that really true?

Smoking and Energy

Cigarettes seem to work as a stimulant—banishing tiredness, improving mood, and stimulating digestion. So what is it about that apparent alarm-clock function of the morning cigarette? Does smoking really help? The stimulant effect of nicotine can be measured: neurotransmitters are released, and EEG tests (measuring brainwave activity) show that brain wave speed increases. ("So it does help! I knew it!") It's true, smokers with low nicotine levels in the morning have less active brain waves than do smokers who've already had their morning fix. However, it's only true up to a point: Smokers who've already smoked that day have EEG activity identical to that of nonsmokers![40] In other words, the nicotine confers no advantage but only resolves the withdrawal symptoms, and with them the morning fatigue. That is, by your smoking away the nighttime withdrawal that is making you lethargic, the morning tobacco hangover, the cigarette just provides the boost that returns you to the normal energy level of a nonsmoker. But energy levels are not all that are low in the morning; mood tends to lag also. Thus, it's no surprise that nonsmokers can seem such pests in the morning. Imagine to yourself for a moment how much nicer it would be to be less fatigued in the morning and be in a better mood, rather than having to smoke your way out of the doldrums first.

Biological Peak

Many people reach their biological performance peak 2 to 3 hours after getting up. That's the point at which one is rested, focused, in a good mood, and ready to perform. Are there any differences here between smokers and nonsmokers? To find out, scientists interviewed strongly addicted smokers, lightly addicted smokers, and nonsmokers every hour about their ability to perform, their subjective activation, and their mood.[41] The result: Very heavy smokers with a high degree of addiction reached their peak activation and mood 3 hours more slowly than did the nonsmokers, with the lightly addicted smokers falling in between. The heavy smokers had the least energy and were in a noticeably worse mood in the mornings, and hence showed greatest improvement after a cigarette. Measured across the day, though, their values remained below the mood levels of the light smokers and non-smokers. Think back to the Fangerström test on pages 55–56. Light smokers haven't yet developed an addiction so strong that they have to smoke themselves out of a low every morning. Some smoke their first cigarette in the afternoon, or even just on certain occasions. But the more addicted to nicotine you become, the earlier in the day you will light that first cigarette. Moreover, between cigarettes over the course of the whole day, you will experience constant and significant fluctuations in mood and energy. It is important that you understand this: Nicotine is not a support, but in fact the cause of these daily ups and downs. The longer and more strongly you depend on this treacherous "ally," the worse the lows become, as well as the more distorted your own self-image. You will come to believe more and more strongly that you are simply inclined to suffer from stress and negative moods. Perhaps it's time to kick the habit and again feel what it's like to be free, in a good mood, and full of energy.

Concentration

"Well, I can certainly concentrate better after having a smoke." "If I feel distracted and agitated, I have a cigarette and am mentally back to normal." Yes, that's how it seems for many people—concentration, stimulation, and smoking go hand in hand. If you've made it through the book this far and feel you're losing concentration, have a smoke now, if you feel it will help. For smokers, a cigarette usually does improve concentration—and I'll explain why in a moment. So, please go ahead. There's no reason to avoid that cigarette right now and I want you to be focused.

Smoke break

Concentration (continued)

Many smokers find it hard that they can no longer smoke in the office. Somehow, those nagging nonsmokers never understood why people smoked in their workplace: to cope with stress and stay focused. Now you are forced to stand outside and suck in a dose of concentration. The prejudice that smokers are always sneaking out just to get away from work isn't fair—but does smoking really improve concentration? And how could you test this?

In a study, smokers were given a series of letters: AA, BB, GH, BBB, CF, JK, HG, UI, KHL. The smokers were instructed that if 3 letters were present in the series (e.g., BBB, KHL), they should be crossed out. Seems simple, doesn't it? Checking several pages of such material under time pressure requires a fair amount of concentration, however.

The smokers were given this test directly after smoking, and again 2, 4, 6, and 24 hours after having last smoked a cigarette.[42] The longer the time since their last cigarette, the less concentrated they were, and the fewer letters they crossed out. It is clearly apparent how quickly performance levels fall, directly in line with nicotine levels.

When the same test was performed with subjects allowed to smoke whenever they wanted, smokers and nonsmokers crossed out the same number of letters. So, you might say, "See, smoking does somehow improve concentration!" And you're right: Smoking does make smokers who are undergoing light withdrawal more focused.

More Nicotine Doesn't Help You Concentrate

Hollywood has shown it a million times: Whenever you see smoking characters working on some difficult task, they light up one after another, as though concentration would get better with every cigarette. For a long time, it was thought that nicotine helped people concentrate. It seems like a logical choice, then, to gain an advantage in concentrating by smoking more. So, does a higher nicotine intake actually make you increasingly focused? That's been tested, too—like this, for example: Smokers were presented with rapid sequences of numbers on a screen, and had to press a button whenever they saw 3 even numbers in a row, such as 888, or 3 odd ones, such as 777.[43] In this way, researchers could test alertness, reaction speed, and concentration. All the smokers had smoked within the previous 45 minutes, so no smoker was suffering from strong nicotine withdrawal. The testing period lasted for 5 minutes, followed by a 10-minute break. During the break, half the test subjects were allowed to smoke, and half were not. The second test run showed no positive effects on alertness, reaction speed, and concentration for the half of the smokers who had ingested additional nicotine. In other words, more nicotine doesn't make you more focused; it just temporarily quells the nervousness caused by withdrawal, which negatively affects concentration. Once that level is reached, no further concentration benefits are shown.

After just 30 minutes, smokers can start to feel declines in their mood. This only starts to affect concentration somewhat later, at the time when restlessness has increased to the point where it overpowers their ability to focus. Thus, in this study, the smokers gained no measurable advantage in the first hour by smoking additional nicotine—but after 2 hours, the withdrawal effects were so strong that their concentration began to fail.

Smoker's Block

Anyone who's ever breathed deeply at an open window can testify to the beneficial effect of oxygen on intellectual performance.

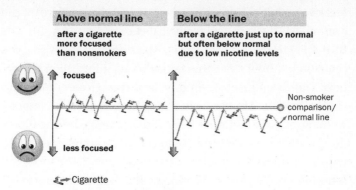

However, if you sit at your desk and smoke one cigarette after another, less and less oxygen is making its way to your brain. Why is that? The carbon monoxide from the cigarettes binds 300 times as strongly to the oxygen transportation mechanism in your red blood cells. The next few hours, as your oxygen is displaced, much too little of it is transported to your brain. Even if nicotine did have some stimulating effect, heavy smokers unquestionably suffer disadvantages due to a lack of oxygen in their brains.

Concentration, Learning, Memory

Do you remember the graph with the normal line? Take another look. Does a smoker exceed the normal line of a nonsmoker in terms of concentration, or not? To really know the answer, one would have to compare nonsmokers, smokers without nicotine deprivation, and smokers deprived of nicotine.

We see the same pattern with which we're familiar from the previous chapter where we looked at stress, stimulation, and pleasure. Once again, smokers not dealing with withdrawal and nonsmokers scored equally well on the test of concentration, whereas smokers undergoing withdrawal fared worse; only after a cigarette break were they able to smoke their way to a normal level of concentration. This is true of the alphabet error tests (AA, BB, GH, BBB, CF, HH, JK, HG, UI, KHL), which demonstrate visual concentration.[44] But it's also true for gathering information that you hear. This listening concentration is of even greater importance in everyday life. Studies have shown that smokers undergoing withdrawal learn and remember auditory verbal information at the same levels as nonsmokers and smoking smokers only once they have smoked and filled up with nicotine.[45] The more concentration varies due to nicotine withdrawal in the course of a day, the greater the overall reduction in performance.

Concentration and Inner Stress

Try to concentrate sometime when you're distracted, when something's under your skin and you're feeling stressed, your stomach is growling with hunger, or you really need to use the bathroom: Try as you might, you can't—if at all, then not very well. It's just the same for smokers with declining levels of nicotine in their blood: The pressure rises, and with it, the tension caused by the lack of nicotine. A general feeling of dissatisfaction, as though something's missing, makes itself felt. The longer you put off getting another cigarette, the more impossible it becomes to concentrate fully on anything, until the only thing on your mind is that next cigarette break.

Mira is a typical example from my stop-smoking seminars. She has to sit constantly through meetings at work where—unlike in the old days—nobody is allowed to smoke. When she's not in meetings, she can hardly leave her office, because there's so much organizing to be done for the meetings. It's torture for her—by the time she's finally able to get away and light a cigarette, she's completely frazzled. The "I like smoking" excuse has its flaws here, too: Looked at in terms of benefits and advantages, the nervous withdrawal cannot be explained logically. Only once the tension is smoked away is it once again possible to be relaxed and concentrated. In the final analysis, rather than battle daily with this constant up-and-down, it's simpler to be a nonsmoker. Nonsmokers can at least concentrate without facing that pressure.

IMPORTANT: It's important to stop lying to yourself that "the cigarette helps me concentrate." That's completely false. The truth is that the cigarette is the reason you can't focus, and it provides only temporary relief from the symptoms of nicotine withdrawal—nothing more. Concentration is not better among nicotine-saturated smokers than among nonsmokers. All that you attain is a normal level of concentration, and for that, you pay with your health—a very high cost indeed. When you escape the vicious cycle of nicotine use, that problem will vanish in just a few weeks. You can make it! And, in the future, when you feel tired and can't concentrate, perhaps you just need to take a little break—like everybody else.

Analyze Your Smoking Behavior

You probably smoke most cigarettes automatically and without being consciously aware of it. Consciously observing your smoking behavior can be very illuminating:

When do you smoke, and at what intervals?

How strong is your smoking urge after the passage of a certain amount of time?

How much do you enjoy a cigarette after a short interval versus after a long one?

What mood are you in when you want to smoke?

Does stress affect your smoking behavior?

When you smoke to feel better or improve your concentration, observe the following:

How long has it been since you last smoked?

If you haven't smoked for 3 or 4 hours, does a single cigarette restore your well-being or concentration? Or do you still want a second dose of nicotine?

Feel free to experiment: If you intentionally smoke another cigarette even when you don't really want to (i.e., you're not trying to "smoke away" your withdrawal symptoms), do you feel better or more focused? Was the cigarette satisfactory, and did it meet your expectations? Or was it insignificant, as you'd smoked too soon after your previous cigarette?

The questionnaire in the book will help you carefully approach these problems. You can also print out the questionnaire from the homepage of the website. It's formatted in such a way that it will fit, folded up, in any pack of cigarettes—one for the road, so to speak.

 CHAPTER 8
link to printable questionnaire

Victory Assured

"Really, I'd prefer to have a simple explanation like, 'This is how you quit.'" Well, easy solutions tend to have a problem. You're enthusiastic about quitting, but quite soon you'll think, "Well, really, I enjoy smoking," and you'll start once more. A little bit of knowledge can be a dangerous thing. All smokers believe smoking brings them some sort of advantage, otherwise they wouldn't keep smoking or picking it up again. Only when you recognize

TIME	SITUATION/ LOCATION	DESIRE TO SMOKE	MOOD	STRESS LEVEL	EXPECTATION OF A CIGARETTE	DID THE CIGARETTE MEET YOUR EXPECTATIONS?
	Examples of triggering situations: Alone, at work, with colleagues, while waiting, while traveling, at home, in your free time, with friends, after eating, with coffee, with alcohol, etc.	0 = ok 1 = medium 2 = strong 3 = must smoke	0 = stable/content 1 = ok 2 = somewhat uneasy/ slightly discontent 3 = not ok	0 = calm/relaxed 1 = somewhat tense/slightly nervous 2 = tense/nervous/ slightly stressed 3 = irritated	1. relaxing 2. improve well-being 3. improve mood 4. reduce discontent 5. reduce stress 6. enjoyment 7. dispel fatigue 8. concentration 9. sociability	0 = not at all 1 = not really 2 = somewhat 3 = entirely

that nicotine addiction has you in its grip, can you break that grip. Great leaders know how to win great victories:

> *If you know neither yourself nor the enemy, you will lose every battle. If you know yourself, and not your enemy, you will suffer a loss for every victory you win. If you know yourself and your enemy, you need not fear the outcome of a hundred battles.*
> —Sun Tzu, *The Art of War*

THE BOTTOM LINE

- ▶ The morning cigarette doesn't give smokers more energy or a better mood than nonsmokers, it just gets them out of the low created by nicotine itself.
- ▶ Energy levels and the ability to concentrate fluctuate strongly in smokers. A low level of nicotine results in concentration problems.
- ▶ Nicotine only improves concentration by temporarily quelling the distracting restlessness caused by nicotine withdrawal. Additional nicotine does not improve alertness, performance, or concentration.
- ▶ In performance tests, smokers attain the normal concentration and performance levels of nonsmokers only by raising nicotine levels in their blood.

9

Stress and Mood

When You Started,
When You're Quitting

Quitting: Renunciation or More Well-Being?

"I worry that if I quit smoking, I may be less content, feel less happy, have less enjoyment, and be more susceptible to stress." That's a typical concern, and again reflects the "smoking as benefit" pattern of thought. The belief that, on some occasions at least, a smoker manages to exceed the normal level of well-being that a nonsmoker has. For this reason, scientists have carefully studied 2 groups of smokers, young people *starting* to smoke and smokers who are *quitting*.

- If smoking were a benefit, young people who started to smoke should feel better, be more content, and have fewer mood swings.
- Smokers who quit should be less happy, less content, and suffer more from stress, because they would no longer enjoy the benefits of smoking, and they would be missing something.

98

Think back to the first cigarettes you smoked as a young person. Did you really think, "Wow, I suddenly feel better!" or "I haven't felt this relaxed in a long time!" or "Cool, this feels great!"? Or did that feeling only develop over time, once you started to "enjoy" smoking? How long does it take to become addicted to nicotine? Or, to put it another way, at what point do young people who begin to smoke "enjoy" smoking? What would you estimate—after 10 packs? 20? What's your answer?

Hooked on Nicotine Checklist—Test Yourself

To answer this question, researchers developed the HONC test for youth. Even if you're no longer an adolescent, answer the following brief questions:

HONC Questionnaire

1. Have you ever tried to quit smoking, but failed?
   Yes ❑   No ❑

2. Do you keep smoking because it's hard to quit?
   Yes ❑   No ❑

3. Have you ever felt as though you were addicted to tobacco?
   Yes ❑   No ❑

4. Have you ever felt a strong desire to smoke?
   Yes ❑   No ❑

5. Have you ever felt as though you really needed a cigarette at a particular moment?
   Yes ❑   No ❑

6. Do you find it difficult not to smoke in places
where smoking is not permitted?
Yes ❏   No ❏

If you have tried to quit, or if you haven't smoked in a while,

7. Have you found it difficult to keep concentrating
because you couldn't smoke?
Yes ❏   No ❏

8. Have you ever felt irritable because you couldn't
smoke?
Yes ❏   No ❏

9. Have you ever felt a strong urge or desire to
smoke?
Yes ❏   No ❏

10. Have you ever felt nervous or restless because
you couldn't smoke?
Yes ❏   No ❏

Nicotine—The Fast Track to Addiction

96,156 young people between the ages of 14 and 15 were given
this questionnaire.[46] Of those surveyed, 24,995 had already exper-
imented with cigarettes. The results are astounding and show
just how quickly you get addicted to nicotine. With every cigarette, the dependence of the young brain deepens. After only a
few cigarettes, more and more young people gave these answers
to the following questions.

"Oh, so many numbers. It's too complicated for me." It's not complicated at all, and quite fascinating: Just read a question and then
read along the arrow, otherwise it's easy to get lost in the numbers.

		How many cigarettes have you already smoked?				
		3–5	6–15	16–25	25–99	>100
Have you ever felt you really needed a cigarette?	Yes	22%	35%	47%	62%	85%

		How many cigarettes have you already smoked?				
		3–5	6–15	16–25	25–99	>100
1. Have you ever tried to quit smoking but did not make it?	Yes	11%	11%	17%	26%	51%

		3–5	6–15	16–25	25–99	>100
2. Do you keep smoking because it is too difficult to quit?	Yes	3%	5%	9%	15%	44%

		3–5	6–15	16–25	25–99	>100
3. Have you ever felt that you were totally dependent on tobacco?	Yes	8%	10%	16%	28%	62%

		3–5	6–15	16–25	25–99	>100
4. Have you ever felt a strong desire to smoke?	Yes	10%	20%	23%	38%	68%

		3–5	6–15	16–25	25–99	>100
5. Have you ever felt like you really needed a cigarette right now?	Yes	22%	35%	47%	62%	85%

How many cigarettes have you already smoked?

	3–5	6–15	16–25	25–99	>100

6. Do you find it hard to not smoke in places where smoking is not allowed?

Yes 9% 11% 17% 29% 58%

When you tried to quit or when you have not smoked for a while:

	3–5	6–15	16–25	25–99	>100

7. Did you find it difficult to concentrate when you were not able to smoke?

Yes 3% 5% 9% 13% 43%

	3–5	6–15	16–25	25–99	>100

8. Did you feel irritable because you could not smoke?

Yes 4% 6% 12% 21% 50%

	3–5	6–15	16–25	25–99	>100

9. Did you have a strong urge or desire to smoke?

Yes 8% 14% 18% 31% 65%

	3–5	6–15	16–25	25–99	>100

10. Did you feel nervous, restless or anxious?

Yes 4% 6% 11% 16% 45%

The Power of Just a Few Packs

Isn´t it amazing how quickly the addiction develops after only a few packs? You wouldn´t believe it without looking at the percentages! Of all the drugs studied, cigarettes are the most addicting. And addiction means that you always smoke to remove feelings of withdrawal! This results in more anxiety, nervousness, and mood swings. A benefit for the psyche? Not really!

Every single cigarette changes the nervous system and steers young brains toward addiction. After only 4 packs, half of all the girls and boys answered yes to 7 out of 10 questions. This means that they are already fully dependent and find it difficult to quit. Even more amazing is that after only 3 to 5 cigarettes, a third of girls and a quarter of boys answered yes to 3 questions regarding addiction. Thus, it does not take years; addiction develops very quickly. You perceive it as "liking to" smoke or "feeling like" smoking and don´t give it a lot of thought. You don't yet understand why, without a cigarette, "something is missing" and why—because of this—you want to continue smoking. So, after a few packs, the "I can quit any time" mantra no longer applies. After 100 smoked cigarettes, half of the adolescents surveyed had already experienced at least one failed attempt to quit. Very soon they no longer smoke because of a misperceived enjoyment, but to eliminate a blank feeling of uneasiness.

Nicotine: A Strong Poison for the Nerves

"Whatever, that can´t be true. How could you become addicted so fast?" The kids' questionnaires clearly show the rapid changes in the brain caused by nicotine. Nicotine acts as a potent neurotoxin directly on the young brain, with rapid and far-reaching changes on the receptors for neurotransmitters and the chemical messenger system as a whole.[47] This was proven in laboratory animal experiments. After the first low dose of nicotine, it is possible to detect immediate and long-lasting adaptation processes in young brains. In the tests, the dose of nicotine was naturally adapted to the body weight of mice and, aside from that, the dose of nicotine was also reduced to one tenth of a mouse-cigarette. Why such a low dose? Young people often take only 3 to 4 drags/hits on a cigarette when they start smoking. The researchers wanted to test whether the lowest levels of nicotine would already lead to changes in the brain. Only a month later, the mouse brains already demonstrated these changes. Has it dawned on you yet? A teenager will smoke one cigarette, then perhaps not another until a buddy offers one several weeks later. But the small changes are still active, and each new cigarette again leaves traces. In children and adolescents, it only takes a few cigarettes to create sustainable changes in the reward center of the brain. Scientists speak of a kind of "sleeper effect" that gradually builds up to addiction. Now it is clear why we see more and more affirmative responses in the questionnaire for HONC-dependence, after only the first cigarettes.

How strongly nicotine shapes the young brain can also be seen in pregnancy. Children are twice as likely to start smoking if their mother smoked during pregnancy—even if she had given up smoking after pregnancy. This is how much the brain of the unborn child is shaped in the long run through early contact with nicotine.

Dependency Despite Smoking Rarely

"Yes, but in my case it took almost a year before I smoked every day." Even if at first you only smoked once a month, it changes the nervous system. Nearly 40% of young smokers reach full dependency before they ever smoke daily.[48] With the increasing changes in the reward center of the brain and because receptors become less and less sensitive to nicotine and even less sensitive to your own neurotransmitters for happiness, the time period after which you need a cigarette to feel content keeps shrinking. Long before that happens, you are already dependent.

The Nicotine Dealer

The strategy and marketing departments of the cigarette industry have long known what scientists have only begun to demonstrate in the last 10 years: Hardly any smokers start after the age of 21, and when they do, they usually remain social smokers and are therefore unprofitable for the smoking industry. Thus, the industry motto is: You have to lure children and young people, with their quickly programmable brains. You also have to make the inhaling of nicotine easier for them with additives, so that they will become addicted quickly. The smoking and thus the industry profits will then automatically increase over the years. This also explains why it is so lucrative for the tobacco companies to distribute free sample packs to teenagers in clubs, or at major events such as concerts. Combining the free samples with a consumer competition is even more clever. A company disclaimer that the participant must be 18 or older circumvents legal restrictions of giving cigarettes to minors. Maybe you encountered these practices when you started smoking! In the United States, these practices are now illegal, but in Europe and in the developing nations they are legal. This is where the tobacco industry experiences growth nowadays. Another way of selling addiction to the young are inexpensive mini-packs or the sale of single cigarettes in third-world countries. The nicotine of each cigarette, which docks on to receptors of the young brain, pays off 100,000 times for the nicotine dealers, who will have a loyal clientele for decades.

In the Clutches of Nicotine from the Start

If the compulsion to smoke starts so quickly, the following is also clear: When we started to smoke, voluntary consumption

was never or only briefly in the foreground, at the very beginning. After just a few cigarettes, we started to smoke mainly to
get us back to feeling "normal"—against the changes already
occurring in the reward center. Of course, for many years we
subjectively "enjoyed" and "liked to" smoke.

It's not easy to digest this news. If instead of enjoyment, the
elimination of withdrawal was in the foreground right from the
start, we are left with the unpleasant feeling of looking back at a
meaningless smoker-life. This will doubtless cause you to be
angry, and you have every right to be! But you, like millions of
other smokers, fell unknowingly into the apparent normality of
nicotine as a teenager. The nicotine trap snapped shut. But that
is in the past. Now, what is the alternative? Business as usual?
Or consciously breaking free from the slavery of nicotine?

Smoking Teens—Frustrated . . . or Frustrated Because of Smoking?

"What is up with the whole rant about addiction among young
people? I want to stop someday . . ." Great, so you want to stop?
Super! But you want to be assured that you will feel better after
quitting and that you won´t miss anything. My initial chal-
lenge was: If smoking is a benefit, then young people would
feel better after they started. Instead, we see that they quickly
become addicted and are soon smoking away nervousness,
restlessness, stress, and mood swings. Surveys show this quite
clearly: Smoking teens have more episodes of depression.

But what came first: Were the youngsters frustrated and
therefore decided to smoke? Or does smoking cause the frustration? One would have to watch young people over many years to
figure this out. And that's exactly what 6 studies involving over
10,000 young people have done. Information about mood and
depression scores were recorded and compared to whether the
subject had started smoking. The results: Young smokers either

had more episodes of depression, or depression set in when they started to smoke.[49] Thus, smoking is not at all a benefit for psychological well-being!

Nicotine Does Not Cure a Bad Mood

There is also the Ping-Pong effect. According to study after study, teenagers with mood swings very often depend on cigarettes and cannot quit.[50] "Perhaps the frustrated teens use nicotine to feel better in the short term. They immediately feel the benefit of smoking," a smoker said to me. Okay—here again we hear the mantra, "Smoking has benefits." Unfortunately, not true! Not a single study has shown that nicotine improves mood swings! Whichever way you look at it, no advantage to one's well-being can be found when one starts to smoke. However, increasing mood swings and stress can already be seen after only a few cigarettes, due to nicotine addiction.

Nicotine Is Not an Antidepressant

Are you familiar with this? Frequent depression and bad moods? Be they teens or adults, there are more smokers with depression than occurs among the nonsmoking population. The cowboy who sits around a campfire and who smokes away his depression does not fit the image that the tobacco industry wants to promote. But one of the main reasons that people continue smoking is to influence mood swings.[51] A cigarette may possibly improve mood caused by the nicotine withdrawal. However, nicotine does not function like an antidepressant drug that one uses for mood improvement. Otherwise, nicotine pills would also improve mood in depressed nonsmokers.[52] No pharmaceutical company has ever applied for the use of nicotine as an antidepressant! Simply put, nicotine does not help nonsmokers.

Nicotine is addictive and only makes the nervous system more irritable and unstable. Someone who already has a predisposition to rapid mood swings, negative feelings, depression, and anxiety will have a heightened sense of the ups and downs of nicotine levels if this substance is administered.

The Most Important Questions of Smokers Who Want to Quit

"Okay. The young are more prone to addiction and we all have more mood swings from tobacco. But I still fear quitting! There will be more stress and less enjoyment. And in any case, I am going to miss smoking!" Did you notice it? There it is again. You have automatically returned to thinking "Smoking is a benefit."

So, what really happens after quitting? If you ask friends and acquaintances about their experiences when quitting, there are more or less 3 ways of telling the story:

- **THE MODEL OF JUSTIFICATION:** "Man, the withdrawal effects were so bad when I quit, I had to start again. Once a smoker, always a smoker. Don't even try it." (Don't let yourself fall into this trap. You now know how smoking works.)
- **THE EPIC HERO:** "It was terrible, but I've made it."
- **THE I-WAS-NEVER-ADDICTED STORY:** "It was quite simple. I just decided to quit."

The problem: Such stories are retrospective and therefore distorted, blurred, or embellished. To get a more truthful assessment, you must survey a smoker right before, during, and several months after quitting. You should survey many smokers, not just a few. Above all, every smoker would have to answer the same questions so you can compare and evaluate them. It is very important that the information be collected neutrally, before the outcome is determined. In homemade smoking surveys, the addicted brain is all too happy to interpret information—especially "facts" tilted in the direction of why it is "too difficult to quit." Information gained from objective studies is therefore more reliable than self-surveys. They clear your head and unmask stereotypes. Why do I put so much emphasis on this? I am not telling you—like other authors—how easy it is to quit. I'll spare you the typical story of Mary, Tom, and John. These stories are a nice read, but they represent isolated cases. I would rather show you what thousands of smokers have actually experienced: solid facts rather than isolated cases. I want to give you a clearer picture of what really happens when smokers quit. This may lessen the anxiety when you do.

Have a Better Life as a Nonsmoker

You will experience the strongest withdrawal symptoms during the first 3 days. This is simply the physical withdrawal. Then it takes about 3 weeks until the changes in the reward center of the brain have switched back to normal. Then you're out of the woods. To prevent these withdrawal symptoms, especially if a heavy smoker, you can use nicotine patches or the drug Champix. Nicotine patches double, and Champix triples, the chances of quitting successfully.

"And then what? I will miss out on something for the rest of my life?" Look at the facts: There are as many ex-smokers as smokers in Germany. 8 out of 10 smokers manage to quit. With so many ex-smokers, you should hear constant lamenting how much poorer their enjoyment of life has become without cigarettes; how hard it is to live every day without nicotine. But, do you hear that? No? Neither do I. Most ex-smokers miss the cigarettes so little that they do not even find it worth mentioning that they were once smokers. They are too busy enjoying the benefits of *not* smoking.

HOW THE PSYCHE BENEFITS FROM QUITTING SMOKING

178 smokers[53]	Withdrawal symptoms will be evaluated after 2, 7, 14, 30, 90, and 180 days.	The withdrawal symptoms of anxiety, low mood, irritability, restlessness, poor concentration, and night waking peaked after 2 days, dropped slightly after 7 days, and after 14 days were at levels prior to smoking cessation. After 30 days, the anxiety, moodiness, irritability, restlessness, and poor concentration were well below the level before quitting!
308 heavy smokers[54]	Stress surveys before and after 1, 6, and 12 months	Smokers who quit indicated having less stress and more self-confidence, were better able to tackle problems, and seemed to be less critical of themselves.
260 smokers[55]	Stress survey before and after 1, 3, and 6 months	Smokers who did not quit had a similar stress level after 1, 3, and 6 months. Smokers who did quit reported a decrease in tension and stress. Important: Before they quit smoking, both groups had the same stress levels. Thus, it was the nicotine cessation that reduced the stress levels.
101 smokers[56]	Anxiety and mood will be evaluated by independent surveys 2 weeks before, 24 hours before, and 1, 2, 3, and 4 weeks later.	Anxiety, negative affect, moodiness, and irritability are greatest on the day one quits smoking, and then improve considerably a week after quitting, to then fall significantly below the baseline established before quitting in the third to fourth week. Anxiety decreases beginning on the first smoke-free day. The climax of anxiety is always with the last cigarette on quitting day.

The Light at the End of the Tunnel

The main message from these studies is that after a brief withdrawal phase, improvement already sets in during the second week. Many smokers fail in the first 2 weeks because they cannot really see whether they will feel better on a day-to-day basis. They get stuck in the dark due to lack of knowledge and doubt, and start to smoke again. Think of it this way: You can handle the flu without problem because you know you will feel better again. This is the same when you quit smoking. You suffer for a short time, instead of having to smoke away the symptoms of withdrawal for the rest of your life.

Are Ex-smokers Less Happy than Smokers?

The quality of life, satisfaction, pleasure, and the psychological well-being of smokers would have to be higher than that of nonsmokers if smoking were a benefit. 9,000 participants (smokers, former smokers, and nonsmokers) were asked 19 key questions about their quality of life.[57] The result: Smoking is associated with lower levels of pleasure and poorer overall quality of life. The smokers fared worse than ex-smokers and nonsmokers.

And what about the feeling of happiness when smokers quit? Are ex-smokers less happy than smokers, because they give up an important source of enjoyment? 879 ex-smokers were interviewed.[58] "Well—those have to be the smokers who did not enjoy smoking as much as I do. I really like to smoke." Precisely for this reason, the ex-smokers were also first asked how much they enjoyed smoking. 28% "had enjoyed it very much," 48% "had enjoyed it," 20% "didn't enjoy it very much," and 3% "had not enjoyed it at all."

Then, 3 significant statements about happiness were assessed: "I feel happier now, compared to the time when I still smoked,"

"I feel just as happy now as when I still smoked," or "I feel less happy compared to the time when I still smoked." Ex-smokers overwhelmingly reported being happier now than when they had been smoking. More than two thirds (69%) reported being happier now than before, 27% said they were as happy, and only 4% claimed to be less happy. You find it surprising to see such results, even though so many had previously "enjoyed" smoking very much? Greater happiness following cessation was not related to prior cigarette consumption or previous perceived enjoyment of smoking. Even if you are a heavy smoker or if you now think you enjoy cigarettes very much, the chances are very high that you will feel more content and happier without smoking.

Let's remain skeptical! Whether the ex-smokers are actually happier than before and why they are happier remains open. It could be the feeling that they are no longer harming themselves; that they are healthier, freer; that they can make it through the day with fewer ups and downs. It could also be self-justification or simply imagination. But one thing is certain: Those who characterized themselves as happier are most likely not unhappier than before, otherwise this would have shown in the results of the study.

The Winning Model for Quitting

When quitting smoking, all smokers only think of the negative. Above all, they shudder at the thought that from now on they will have less pleasure in life, and they will not be able to control stress and their mood. This again goes hand in hand with the mantra, "Smoking as a benefit." If it were a psychological advantage, one would naturally miss something. But smoking offers no benefit for the psyche, and I think I've proved that to you in detail. You lose nothing when you quit—you only gain. And what could be better than getting your freedom back and being able to feel normal and happy without a cigarette.

THE BOTTOM LINE

- ▶ If smoking were a benefit, then young people should feel better and more satisfied when they start smoking, and smokers should be less happy, less satisfied, and more stressed after quitting.
- ▶ Young people are addicted after only a few packs. They will then soon smoke to eliminate a restless, dissatisfied feeling. As a result, they experience more depressive moods once smoking has begun.
- ▶ Nicotine is not an antidepressant; otherwise it would have long since been an approved drug.
- ▶ On the contrary: Depression and mood changes are a result of nicotine and increase through nicotine considerably.
- ▶ Smokers who quit report after just a short time that they experience less stress, more stable moods, and more satisfaction.
- ▶ Overall, 96% of ex-smokers feel happier than or as happy as they were before smoking.

10

Interview with Prof. Parrott— Smoking and the Mind

PROF. ANDREW C. PARROTT IS AN expert, worthy of his title. Not only has he published 300 articles on all types of psychoactive drugs, Prof. Parrott has also published pioneering studies on the psychological and emotional effects of nicotine dependence, and is an internationally renowned authority on the subject. It was important to me to interview him for you. So I flew to Cardiff, Wales, and was happy that he had reserved half a day for our conversation.

Andreas Jopp: *How did you end up working on nicotine?*

Andrew Parrott: I worked for several years analyzing the psychopharmacological effect of medications before I started to research the effects of nicotine. I was at the University of East London for 17 years, and the main drug I started looking at was nicotine . . .

AJ: *In one of your studies, you examined the mood right before and after smoking. Usually, smokers only see the direct benefits of smoking. In your studies, it is much more exciting to see what happens in between 2 cigarettes.*

AP: Well, the first few years of my nicotine research, I fit very neatly into the model of "nicotine increasing cognition and improving mood." I had no problem with that at the time, until I submitted a study that was picked apart by its reviewer. While I assumed that nicotine improved mood and cognition, the reviewer said I needed to be more circumspect in that and needed to rephrase the discussion to say it may well improve mood and cognition although that was yet to be discerned. So, like most reviewers' comments, you find them extremely annoying, so I had to edit the discussion to fit in, but it really got the seed of doubt going. I found that nobody was really looking at this question, if nicotine is actually improving mood and cognition or not. I had to test that properly. So I had the idea of getting people to rate the moods before and after each cigarette to see the effects of the cigarette, but then crucially ask them to rate the mood just before they had the next cigarette. The crucial aspect of that study is how the mood is going to change in the end, from the previous cigarette to the beginning of the next one. So then you can actually plot this time and profile what's happening between cigarettes, which nobody had done before. This really changed my views on nicotine, when I looked at the findings.[59]

AJ: *So you were surprised by the extent of changes in mood . . .*

AP: I can remember my feelings, when I was processing the data on the computer and the results were

Interview with Prof. Parrott—Smoking and the Mind

115

coming out and I was just staring at these graphs as the scales fell in front of my eyes and suddenly everything fit. And it is one of these dramatic moments for scientists, when you suddenly realize it all fits into place. I said, yes, this is a crucial aspect with deprivation, in that you saw dotted lines between cigarettes in particular. When people haven't smoked for 2 hours, you've got a big drop. But even if you haven't smoked for 30 minutes, you have a drop in moods and a smaller gain on the next cigarette.

AJ: *These mood changes are usually very small. A smoker may only get a feeling of emptiness and that he would like to smoke to get rid of it. The relief is felt as pleasure. Is that the real danger of nicotine as a highly addictive drug—that you don't recognize it as such?*

AP: This is the essence of the problem, I think. If you light up a cigarette and have 2 or 3 inhalations, you'll get a rapid mood gain stroke normalization; but if you're not smoking for 30 or 40 minutes, your mood loss will be so subtle you won't attribute it to nicotine deprivation. You'll just think, "Well, I haven't smoked in a while; I probably just need one." But you won't say that it is nicotine. And this is one of the problems with being a smoker: Over time, smoking makes you more nervous, makes you more moody, makes your moods more liable. Again that occurs over months and years, so if you've been a smoker for 1 or 2 years, you're slightly more moody, irritable, easily upset. This altered baseline has become part of your personality and you now label yourself as slightly easily upset, easily stressed, and if there is one thing you think, it is that a cigarette will calm you down. So your attributions of yourself as a person changes very slowly over time, just as your attributions of mood loss during abstinence changes. This is one of the key properties of mood with nicotine. You need to realize what it's doing to you. It's very subtle.

AJ: *If you attribute the decreasing stress resistance to your personality after only a few years, what do you do after 20 or 30 years of smoking? After such a long time, you can't remember how relaxed you once were. Logically, you then have the impression that a cigarette would calm you down and that you don't want to give that up.*

AP: Yes, and you think of nervousness as part of you, without realizing that it is caused by being nicotine dependent.

AJ: *Another ground-breaking study examines whether smoking is a real gain in well-being or not.*[60] *Do smokers in the short term experience more pleasure and better moods than nonsmokers do?*

AP: Well, you've certainly got more variable mood and many smokers will say that smoking is giving them a mood lift, which it is. The big problem is the withdrawal. This is probably making smokers more moody and leading them to the mood vacillations. So a smoker over a day will have more mood changes. The peak moods are probably comparable to those of normal nonsmokers, but the lows are well below normal. The big problem is really in between cigarettes, when moods of smokers will be worse. So in terms of daily experiences, a smoker will have more gradual mood losses and more rapid mood reversals, which they will call "gains." So, you can see why it is an attractive drug and you can see why people attribute positive things to these "gains."

Interview with Prof. Parrott—Smoking and the Mind

117

AJ: *Despite these downward fluctuations, one could always say, "Yes, but the mood is improving yet again and perhaps the last good mood was a bit above the normal feeling of a nonsmoker. Maybe that's the kick I need."*

AP: What you can say is that the average mood of the day is never better than that of a nonsmoker. So, there are never real mood gains. You see, these days, they are putting more restrictions on smoking so you can't light up whenever you need a mood lift. So you're bound to get smokers who clearly are suffering more than in former days, when people could light up anywhere.

AJ: *So, after smoking, smokers tend to feel less nervous and tense and more relaxed and calm. Does smoking reduce stress? Or does it build up more stress?*

AP: Well, over the day, the relaxation is probably not very long lasting. What's probably happening is that 10 to 20 minutes after that last cigarette, your nervousness is already starting to build up ever so slightly. Probably it's very difficult to monitor, but then after about 30 minutes, if you are a regular smoker, you will notice it more and start being dissatisfied, irritable, and ill-tempered, and if you are in a very long meeting—2 hours, 3 hours—you can really see the pain for smokers. They get short-tempered. I was in a meeting where the chairman was a heavy smoker and he kept on calling coffee and smoking breaks, because he was getting more and more irritable over time. You could see his nervousness building up. No one else in the meeting was a smoker. So, it was a very disruptive meeting.

AJ: *Do you think that smokers smoke because of a higher susceptibility to stress, or are they more nervous because they smoke?*

AP: I think there is a dynamic interaction between the two. If you are a naturally emotionally labile person who is naturally nervous and you take up smoking, I think you'll rapidly become a heavy smoker who suffers without nicotine and who gains a lot through mood reversal, so you've got the biggest zigzag or vacillation. In the study with the 105 participants, those who reported using cigarettes as a way of stress control were the heaviest smokers. They were also the smokers with the greatest use of nicotine for alertness control. So, they suffered the most stress from nicotine.

If you're low in neuroticism, you won't have so much mood vacillation with nicotine and then you'll often follow a different pattern of smoking. You'll probably become more of a light social smoker—it will take you longer to become a heavy dependent smoker, and if you're lucky, you may never become that. You may manage to remain a light smoker over time. I think you've got the same with depression: If you are a naturally depressed person, you'll follow the same pattern, where you'll get more depressed in-between cigarettes, but get a better mood lift when you light up. This, I think, explains why depressed people are overrepresented among smokers, why they are often heavy smokers. Overall, these highs and lows are reduced by smoking cessation.

AJ: *We have not yet talked about concentration and mental performance . . .*

AP: If you look at the cognitive side of smokers over the day, they seem to be normal—they are not impaired. So, whereas their stress levels are worse than normal, their cognition isn't as long as the nervousness due to low nicotine levels is not excessive.

We know that nicotine is improving cognition for a short moment when a smoker lights up. But we also know that it is deteriorating between cigarettes. Cognition may be speaking above average for a few minutes, but then it is gradually deteriorating and getting below the average level of a nonsmoker, as your abstinence is increasing and distracting you. The big weakness of the nicotine in cognition literature is that most of it doesn't take into account the abstinence problem. Most of nicotine research is looking at short-term acuteness studies focusing on positive gains post-nicotine. What they really need to do is focus equally upon the deteriorating period after that, which they never seem to do.

AJ: *Smokers have increasing difficulties because smoking is banned in offices. So over the day, you will have longer periods between cigarettes. I remember you had a study where you measured the effect on mental performance with increasing time of abstinence. The longer the time between cigarettes, the less able the smoker was to concentrate in performance tests.*

AP: Yes. Little was known about the course of nicotine withdrawal symptoms. How quickly do these symptoms appear? So we measured task performance but also stress, irritability, and mood after 2 and 6 hours of abstinence. In terms of cognition you could see that already after 2 hours of abstinence, a drop in task performance. In another study we looked at the hassles, cognitive failures, and daily uplifts of deprived smokers, nondeprived smokers, and nonsmokers.[61] Nicotine did not generate any real psychobiological gains or advantages. Instead, dependent smokers need regular hits of nicotine just to feel normal.

AJ: *Many smokers say, "I just can't go through my day without a cigarette." Do smokers have a real gain on arousal and alertness with nicotine?*

AP: I think you've probably got a slight gain on nicotine while smoking. But after 10 minutes, your arousal and alertness is going to be rapidly declining. So, over the day, the arousal level of a smoker is going up and down, just as the stress level does. And the arousal, the alertness of a smoker is actually worse over the day than that of a nonsmoker, in terms of self-rating. So, when you are a heavy smoker, you certainly need a cigarette to get your arousal system into gear in the morning. The basic problem is your arousal will be going up and down over the day and you'll be suffering again and again without nicotine. Then you need to light up just to get this "gain." So basically the nicotine dependency is causing your arousal to fluctuate, to vacillate over the day, and your arousal suffers because you are a smoker.

AJ: *What changes do you see when smokers quit?*

AP: Well, the first thing to say is that about half of smokers find quitting easier than they thought. And about half of smokers say it is very difficult. I think those that find it easier are those who have less of the mood vacillations. Those who find it most difficult are the groups that have mood swings and get depressed easily. So, the people with the strongest abstinence problems and thus the strongest gains on nicotine restoration statistically may have the greatest problems in quitting. On the other hand, those smokers will gain the most on the psychological side once they are nonsmokers and off

Interview with Prof. Parrott—Smoking and the Mind

121

the vacillations that you have with nicotine. So, one message to smokers is: Try quitting, it may be easier than you think. The other is that heavy smokers may feel the strongest gains over time when stopping.

So, many smokers will report, "Well, I'd expected to be terrible and miserable and I was a bit irritable, a bit miserable, a bit short-tempered, but not as bad as I thought and I found quitting not too difficult." The average smoker will suffer from irritability, a short temper, poor memory, poor concentration, and moodiness. But all of this is for a limited time.

AJ: *What's happening when you get over this short withdrawal period? It would be logical that ex-smokers have less mood, stress, and arousal change . . .*

AP: The study by Cohen and Lichtenstein[62] reported on smoking cessation and how the moods improve. That was a very important study replicated by lots of other scientists. The mood was getting better after 2 weeks of cessation, even better after a month, and still better after 6 months. So, the message for smokers is: Quit and your mood will get better; you will become less moody, less stressed; you will grow calmer each day, less dependent upon nicotine, less moody, less depressed; there is a whole range of gains that you will have. It also creates greater self-efficacy, because you will be doings things without the crutch of nicotine.

AJ: *So, why do many relapse after 6 months?*

AP: Smokers often relapse due to social pressure. They say things like, "I realized that I wasn't that dependent, therefore, when someone offered me a cigarette I thought, 'I'll light up because I can quit easily,'" and now they're back as a smoker.

Lots of relapses are the result of stress. When people are faced with a major life stress, bereavement, loss of job—that's one key time when they relapse. And then, many relapse in social situations that involve alcohol. With alcohol, your inhibitions will be reduced, your cognitive thinking is less clear than it should be. Other people are lighting up around you; you're then likely to have "just one cigarette," and when nicotine starts to leave your body, you want another one.

AJ: *The combination of alcohol and cigarettes is very typical . . .*

AP: Alcohol and nicotine counteract each other. Basically, alcohol is a sedative drug, and the only drug that has been shown to counteract that is nicotine. What seems to be happening is if you drink alcohol, your sedation is going down, and with smoking nicotine, you can modulate your alertness.

So, my advice is that if you are trying to quit smoking, avoid for a while areas where there are other smokers— and avoid alcohol. When you go out, tell others not to offer you a cigarette. Prewarn them. Say you're not going to be happy if they offer you a cigarette and you don't want them to smoke in front of you; you don't want them to say that they are going out for a cigarette and you are sure you don't want one. This is a classic way in which people relapse—in a social environment, when inhibitions are reduced through alcohol.

AJ: *What is the best day to stop and how do you handle relapses in general? You have conducted studies with women . . .*

AP: Well, I think the worst time would be premenstrually. Again, this is fairly common sense. So, getting earlier in the cycle, midcycle, is the best time to stop. Then, let's suppose you have got strong premenstrual symptoms; let's suppose you do relapse in those few days—that isn't to say you failed. It means that you relapsed in those few days. So, those may be the 4 days where you smoke a few cigarettes—that's fine; that is a part of life. Now quit again. Then, suppose you manage to quit again for another 20 days, but then during the next premenstrual period you again relapse—again accept that, but then move on. What you find is the third time, you probably won't need more than 1 or 2 cigarettes; in the fourth cycle, you may be able to go through it cigarette free. If you are trying to quit, you are succeeding in quitting, then you relapse due to whatever; it could be a premenstrual period or it could be a stressful moment in your life. This is fine, accept that, you've done that, but it doesn't mean you are a failure. It means you have a few cigarettes, and so go back to baseline and quit again. Don't think, "Oh my God, I've had 4 cigarettes during my premenstrual period—that means that I am terrible, that means I cannot quit, that means I might as well carry on smoking."

123

AJ: *How to handle relapse is just as important for men . . .*

AP: Well, most smokers who do quit, do have slips. So the question is, how do you take that? And I think the message is, if you do relapse, don't use that to label yourself as a failure. Say, "Okay," accept it like your football team: Your football team loses—it isn't the end of the world. You go on from there!

AJ: *Why is the method of quitting smoking all at once so much better from a psychological point of view then to reduce the [number of] cigarettes?*

AP: If you reduce your consumption, you are still addicted to nicotine but you are not getting the mood gains. So, you are suffering greater withdrawal in-between cigarettes over longer periods. Let's suppose that instead of smoking a cigarette every hour, you smoke a cigarette every 3 hours. You cut down from 10 cigarettes a day to 5 cigarettes a day. What you are suffering is longer periods without nicotine. You are also getting stronger mood gains each time you are lighting up, so the nicotine in the cigarettes is becoming more reinforcing. You are suffering the worst of both worlds. You are suffering more abstinence, which will make you moodier, your cognition is worse, your mood states are worse every day, but also each time you have a cigarette, you think you get a big gain. So my recommendation is always: Don't cut down. Quit! If you quit, it is a decision—you are getting rid of nicotine, and cutting down is not a decision to get rid of nicotine, which is another crucial factor. You've got to decide. That is the key thing. If you don't make that decision, nothing much can follow. Do some reading realizing how nicotine works, and once you've got that fully on board, it's pretty easy to quit. And you will find that cessation becomes easier over time. So within a month, you should be a lot better; and in 3 months, you will be a lot better still; in 6 months, even better, and you will maintain that. But you need to take this decision not to use nicotine. The cessation period will be far easier if you simply quit. You'll have a few crappy days, and possibly a few crappy weeks, but the gains from that brief period of total cessation are far better. I guess the main message from my research would be that your life should be better psychologically: You should be less stressed, less depressed, calmer. So look for those benefits and get them.

11

The Power of Conditioning

Your Smoking Pattern

"I do not smoke only when my nicotine levels drop, or when I feel light withdrawal. I enjoy smoking 2 or 3 cigarettes with my coffee, when I am on the phone for a long time, during the commercial breaks while watching TV, after dinner, with beer, when others smoke, and when I go out with friends. Just like that." Smoking as a relief from withdrawal explains only a part of the cigarettes you smoked. There is a second smoking pattern: the conditioned cues. The main reason behind your dependence on nicotine is its persistent linkage to specific situations and cues that cause you to smoke. What is behind these cues? Why do smokers automatically and unconsciously reach for a cigarette when drinking coffee or a beer at the pub? No nonsmoker was ever under the impression that coffee tastes better with a cigarette. Go sit in a café and watch a smoker for a while. You can count to 10: As soon as the coffee is on the table . . . 1–2–3 . . . by the latest at 10 . . . a cigarette has been lit. This has little to do with pleasure, but it happens on autopilot and reflexively.

What causes this reflex-like behavior? Nicotine triggers the release of the neurotransmitter dopamine. With dopamine, certain behaviors are firmly established, or—as it is called—conditioned. Nature wants to reward good and vital behaviors, such as eating and sex, so that these will be executed instinctively. When you smoke, under the influence of dopamine, a lot of situations and occasions are linked to a fixed smoking behavior. Increasingly over time, situations where you use nicotine become a direct trigger for smoking. And this happens regardless of whether you need a cigarette at this very moment to raise the nicotine level again. It happens "just like that," as the smoker said above. An example: You go out with friends and have fun. No nonsmoker needs a cigarette in this situation. But as a smoker, you have time and again established an inseparable link in your head between going out and smoking. The same is true of smoking after sex. Whoever came up with the idea to smoke after sex, when you could also just doze off? Only a smoker. Many smokers ask themselves all their lives why they smoke in different situations, almost obsessively. The only reasons given: "It's just such a habit," or "I just enjoy it." But what's so pleasurable about drawing smoke into the lungs? Let's take a look behind the scenes, to learn why so many situations encourage smoking.

The Power of Everyday Life

Cigarettes are a socially accepted drug. The result: No other drug is used to such an extent in daily life as nicotine is. It is in this way that nicotine gets the chance to condition the smoker to smoke in many situations, through repeated dopamine releases.

These fixed-condition trigger situations make us continue to smoke automatically.[63] The great fear of all smokers who have linked many everyday situations with smoking is, of course, that they believe they would never be able to enjoy these nice situations without a cigarette. An evening at the pub without smoking, for example, is hard to imagine—because this linkage had become a permanently learned behavior pattern.

Now to you: In what situations do you always smoke?

1. _____

2. _____

3. _____

4. _____

5. _____

6. _____

7. _____

8. _____

What Exactly Is Conditioning?

Have you ever heard of the Pavlovian reflex? Ivan Pavlov, a Russian Nobel Prize winner, researched involuntary reflexive behavior. One of his experiments was to ring a bell when he fed dogs. After some time, the dogs made an association between the bell and food. Then, when the bell rang but no food was given, the dogs came anyway, drooling. Hungry or not! It was very hard to unlearn this behavior again. "But, Mr. Jopp, that's obvious: That was about eating. And I am neither a dog, nor do I drool. I just enjoy a cigarette with coffee." Well, I just wanted to first explain the Pavlovian reflex to you. Let's take the experiment one step further. And, we are not talking about you now. Let us look at some nicotine-dependent mice and see just how they deal with nicotine and well-learned situations.

How Mice Learned to Become Nicotine-Dependent

In a famous study,[64] individual mice were trained to desire nicotine. In the "I-am-going-to-give-myself-a-nicotine-fix-now-box," the mouse could choose between 2 levers: one lever with a saline solution, and one with nicotine. If the nicotine lever was pressed, it emitted a light signal and there was an instant nicotine infusion via an intravenous tube. The light turned off when the nicotine infusion was complete. It didn't take the mouse long to be interested only in the nicotine lever. The mouse brain also stored the closely linked stimuli: Light signal = nicotine-dopamine fix. After 2 to 3 weeks, this led to very reliable drug-seeking behavior.

By now, for the mouse, it was the most natural thing in the world that when the pleasant light came on, it could treat itself to some nicotine, so as to enjoy everything together. At this point, the desire for nicotine and the light simply belonged together. However, the box was then reset: When over several weeks, the behavior had been learned and the link had been established, the nicotine in the lever on the left was replaced by a salt solution. Each time the mouse pressed the lever and the light came on, now it got only saline. Too bad. In the beginning, the mouse still showed fully purchasing behavior, often desperately pushing on the lever—just as I desperately used to bang on cigarette vending machines when they were stuck or out of order. After 12 days, the withdrawal was over and the mouse showed little interest in pressing the lever despite its activating the light signal. The behavior was completely unlearned again. It took a while but it worked.

Now, the unlearned behavior was put to the test by giving the mouse a preinfusion of nicotine. Nevertheless, it did not press the lever for replenishment—even when the light appeared. Not interested. Thus the nicotine-lever/light conditioning had become completely unlearned. The mouse had quit.

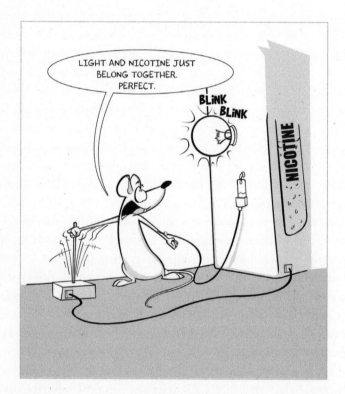

CONDITIONED AND COMPLETELY UNLEARNED AGAIN

2–3 WEEKS OF CONDITIONING ON NICOTINE + LIGHT SIGNAL	12 DAYS UNLEARNING WITH LIGHT SIGNAL	TEST WHETHER THE BEHAVIOR IS UNLEARNED
Mice learn to connect the nicotine lever and light signal. Light signal = dopamine fix is firmly learned after a few weeks.	Mice press lever with light signal, but receive only saline. After 10–12 days, the rodents are over the withdrawal and they are not interested in pressing the lever, even with the light signal.	Mice receive a nicotine injection but still have no interest in pressing the lever, despite the drug. Also, the nicotine injection + light signal does not motivate them to press the lever for additional nicotine. The behavior has been completely unlearned. The withdrawal process has been successful.

Incomplete Deconditioning and the Addiction Memory

"Okay. So you can also unlearn something. I don't see the point yet. What does that have to do with the lights?" Exactly. That belongs to the second experiment. Then you will understand why, even if you are physically off nicotine, you still respond to certain key situations with a strong urge to smoke and even have feelings of withdrawal. That's what conditioning is all about. That's what makes nicotine such a powerful drug. The conditioning triggers us to constantly smoke in certain situations and makes us continue to smoke without understanding why. During cessation, these conditioning cues must be unlearned one by one.

In the second experiment, the nicotine-dependent mice again unlearned the fixed drug-seeking behavior by receiving a saline infusion when pressing the lever, *but without the light's coming on* during this infusion. (Remember: The light went on whenever

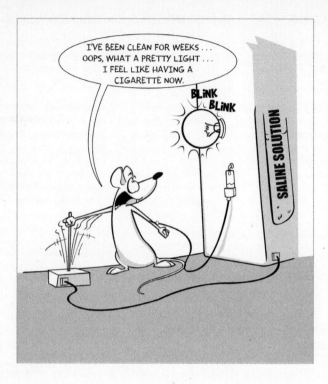

the nicotine solution was given.) Thus the light signal was not unlearned. It stays psychologically linked to the nicotine infusion. After 12 days, the lever pressing was fully unlearned—the mice were clean, the physical withdrawal was done. Even when receiving a nicotine injection, the mice did not return to the old behavior of pressing the lever. The withdrawal process was actually complete, but . . .

Now comes the coffee signal . . . *eh?* . . . Oh, I meant the light signal, of course, which conditioned the rodents with the help of dopamine. And what happened? Bang: The mouse immediately pressed the right nicotine lever—and not just once but push,

push, push, again and again, with the same fierce perseverance as before. Even though the mice were no longer physically addicted to nicotine!

The mice continued this for days, until they finally learned: Light signal = only saline. Only then was the persistent nicotine-light-provision-signal unlearned. A "habit" can be turned off much faster. Pressing the lever 2 or 3 times, the matter would have been done with. It is exactly these persistent smoking triggers that not only give mice, but every human smoker in many situations, such a strong desire to smoke, and we have to unlearn these signals individually.

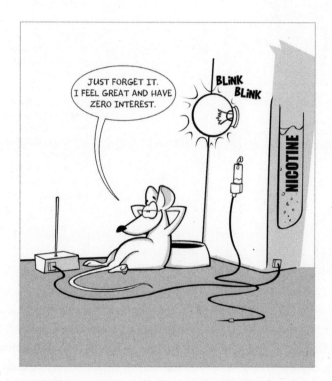

CONDITIONED BUT NOT COMPLETELY UNLEARNED

2–3 WEEKS OF CONDITIONING OF NICOTINE + LIGHT SIGNAL	12 DAYS OF UNLEARNING WITHOUT LIGHT SIGNAL	TEST WHETHER THE BEHAVIOR IS UNLEARNED
	Mice press the lever to get nicotine but receive only saline. After 10–12 days, there is little interest to press the lever.	GROUP 1 mice are tested whether they are "clean" and then receive a nicotine injection in advance. Nevertheless, the mice do not press the nicotine lever to receive more.
		GROUP 2 mice are not dependent anymore and only get a light signal. They press the nicotine lever immediately. Even when they now only receive saline, it takes days until the light signal no longer triggers provision behavior and is finally unlearned.

Enjoyment or Conditioning?

The effect of tobacco as a drug is not a great experience compared to the effects of other drugs. Nicotine is a total loser, based on its very modest mood-altering effects. It is hard to explain why it is so difficult for many smokers to quit smoking, until one considers that the reason cigarettes are so addictive is that the conditioning of nicotine is coupled with so many everyday situations that trigger the desire to smoke. I always thought smoking was part of my lifestyle and that I voluntarily decided to smoke in this or that situation. But— let's be honest—we smoke very few cigarettes deliberately. Most cigarettes are smoked reflexively, conditioned by smoke triggers. After dinner, in the pub, with friends, when others smoke or alcohol comes into play . . . we begin to drool like Pavlov's dogs for the nicotine kick. The mice experiments show how powerful the conditioning of nicotine can be. The mice have never even seen a cigarette advertisement. To want nicotine when receiving a light signal—"just because it goes together"—that is a direct conditioning of a key stimulus by nicotine. It demonstrates how things that have absolutely nothing to do with each other can become linked together. And for the mice, the withdrawal of the conditioned light signal lasts as long as the actual physical withdrawal!

"Great . . . now you have brought me down to the level of a mouse and I'm really pissed." This was not my intention. I want to show you how reliably the drug nicotine can link (condition) certain behaviors to certain everyday situations. It is what it is, whether mouse, or human: The more everyday situations have been conditioned with smoking cigarettes, the more automatic smoking timers you have. Most smokers aren't even aware of this. What we see is, "Ah, the coffee," and already have a cigarette in our hand. Only when asking smokers to shortly reflect on every cigarette do they become aware of this automated action. And then the only tangible reason for the smoker is, "I just wanted a cigarette." In fact, no smoker knows exactly why he or she has this programmed desire to smoke. The experiment with the light signal shows how this desire to smoke has been conditioned as an automatic reflex.

These triggers do not only cause the desire to smoke. They can also trigger feelings of deprivation and the typical craving for cigarettes if we do not give in to the urge, or when we are quitting smoking. The good news: You can get rid of all this learned stimuli. First, determine your personal smoke triggers. The best way to do this is to use the list on page 128.

Drooling on Smoking Triggers

Of course, triggering situations were not only tested with mice, but also with smokers.[65] For example: When photos were shown in which, somewhere in the image, someone was smoking or where someone prepares to smoke a cigarette, smokers reacted with an increased desire to smoke. In the tests, it didn't matter whether the subjects had not smoked for a while (lower nicotine levels) or they had smoked a short time before (higher nicotine levels). Both groups responded with the same desire to smoke. They immediately began to "drool." All smokers have stored many of these smoking cues, which "just happen" to make them smoke. In ex-smokers and nonsmokers, these key attractions do not trigger this "drool" feeling.

Unlearned Is Unlearned

IMPORTANT: When you quit, there are 2 time periods: The end of physical dependence is achieved within 2 to 3 weeks, and then it's about unlearning the smoke triggers, which can cause the classic relapses. We can still learn something from the mice: The mice couldn't care less no matter how much the light flickers, once the conditioning is unlearned. Just as no nonsmoker would ever get the idea to smoke on this or that occasion. Nonsmokers do not notice these smoke triggers at all, because they are not conditioned to them. New ex-smokers, however, are sometimes still aware of them. Still, these situations trigger less and less cravings. And after a while, the triggers are no longer perceived!

Once your programming is unlearned, you will be able to enjoy soccer, beer, and friends without wasting a thought on a cigarette. Just like every nonsmoker. After a while, you are cured of the brainwashing by the nicotine. Welcome to life outside the cigarette pack.

Why Not Just Use Neurotransmitter Blockers?

The scientists behind the mice experiments are not the only mice tamers.[66] [67] [68] A variety of experiments showed the amazing power of conditioning and how difficult it is to break free of an addiction. But it is always possible! The pharmaceutical industry was hoping to find substances that would reduce the desire to smoke in key situations. Neurotransmitter blockers can actually reduce this reflexive behavior to key stimuli.[69] [70] But do we really have to manage everything with the help of drugs? The research made one thing clear: Nicotine has conditioned our behavior with key stimuli via neurotransmitters. This linking of key stimuli is the main reason why we smoke on so many occasions "just like that," why we miss smoking if we resist the urge, why we continue to smoke without a logical explanation, and also why we develop such a strong dependence on nicotine. These are the "smoking traps." Smokers are capable of reprogramming themselves to not react to the situations of everyday life that trigger them to smoke.

Conditioning Is No Habit

"I have always known: I'm a habit-smoker." Smokers perceive the "at any time" and "just like that" cigarettes as habit-cigarettes. However, conditioning is no habit. A habit is something you can change easily. Just as driving on the right or left side of the road. With a habit you do not have the strong urge to drive on the right side again while you are driving on the left side. A desire that triggers obsessive thinking "right right right" and that you will never again enjoy driving if you cannot "immediately" drive on the right side again. The reason for this: conditioning is anchored in the same part of the brain that also encourages vital life-preserving behaviors, such as eating and sex. Only: Your life does not depend on smoking! Although it does feel like that during the acute "I-must-smoke-*now*" panic.

For many smokers, the prospect of life without cigarettes is scary and hardly conceivable. However, any twisted perception of the dire necessity or inevitability of smoking can be altered by critically looking at the facts and reality: Smoking is not vital to survival. You must only undo the conditioning, the brainwashing. Deliberately. With patience. With farsightedness. You now see through these drug-induced magic tricks and will no longer fall for them.

The Psychological Dependence of the Social Smoker

Oliver came to one of my seminars because he did not succeed in quitting smoking entirely. For years he smoked only 3 cigarettes a day, without ever having the feeling that he had to smoke more. But at social occasions, he turned on full blast and always smoked 1 to 2 packs in an evening. He just couldn´t explain this and began to avoid such situations. He had already made 5 attempts to quit. Most smokers would like to be social smokers like Oliver, or think they are. But only 10% of smokers actually fall into this extraordinary group of smokers. Although some smokers can force themselves to smoke very little, they suffer because their brain is accustomed to more nicotine. Social smokers, however, have no feelings of deprivation outside of the fixed, learned smoking situations. This low physical dependence might be genetic. In any case, Oliver could neither stop smoking nor explain this obsessive smoking pattern. As a youngster, Oliver always felt uneasy with others, and felt more confident and adult with a cigarette in his hand. In addition, he wanted to belong. This behavior was conditioned very strongly by nicotine and became a typical trigger situation. Although he is much more confident today, the old conditioning remains a fixed behavior. Shortly after our meeting, he managed to smoke his last cigarette.

Deconditioning Yourself—Your Victory over the Pavlovian Reflex

The conditioned key stimuli can be situations, such as talking on the phone, waiting, trying to concentrate, being alone, after eating, after sex, while watching TV, or drinking coffee or alcohol. It could also be a social occasion, such as meeting a friend with whom you have always smoked together. Or a specific location, such as a doorway, a balcony, or your "smoking couch," may become a trigger. Emotional events are also key stimuli: stress, bad moods, negative affect, which you thought to moderate by smoking. One of the strongest smoking cues is other smokers: You sit on a terrace. No one smokes. Then someone lights up a cigarette and in no time, 3 to 4 other smokers have a cigarette in their hand. Just like that. Situations, places, people, emotional situations, and other smokers—for years you have conditioned these with nicotine as a smoking trigger. You must experience each of these key situations several times without lighting a cigarette. Over time, you will have unlearned all of these triggers. Within a year, there will still be a few events, such as New Year's Eve or meeting with smoking friends you rarely see, to which your same conscious resistance to smoking should apply. And then all the stimuli will be deconditioned. Be patient with the somewhat ponderous brain. It can be trained. Definitely.

"Why does it take that long?" Once more: Conditioned behavior is not a habit. Your mind's reward center, where these fixed triggers are stored, is stubborn, tenacious. Situations must be experienced several times by the reward center as being equally satisfactory without nicotine as formerly with it, until this new behavior is finally saved in a new neural circuit. Remember: Perhaps from the age of 12 you have conditioned a very different behavior to each nicotine trigger, thousands of times. 3 cups of coffee per day with the nicotine drug as a behavioral reinforcer makes about 10,950 coffee-conditioning units in 10 years. Thus, sometime later, coffee itself starts to trigger an immediate impulse to smoke. Another example is to counter stress with a cigarette. 10,000 stress-nicotine conditioning units later, it will become second nature for you to smoke in these situations, instead of looking for other forms of stress release as nonsmokers have. This also means new and better behaviors that work just as well as the knee-jerk response of lighting up must now be found and tried. So give yourself some time.

"I won't be able to take it. I will most definitely get weaker after each temptation that I am trying to control." On the contrary: Every situation in which you have not smoked will make you stronger and is a victory! You already know my approach, that I don´t use untested statements, as are found in other how-to books.

So, here are the facts if resisted temptation challenges your self-control: By means of a mobile device, 309 smokers reported 11,176 resisted temptations.[71] The astonishing result: The more often they recently resisted tempting situations, the lower their risk of future relapses. Actually, it is logical: Each temptation serves as a training session to recondition your brain to make its own decisions again. Therefore, once again: Any situation in which you used to but now have not smoked makes you stronger and is a victory! Each success will give you inspiration and courage for the next. After just a few weeks, you will need fewer of these training sessions.

Think of it with a bit of farsighted humor. You will probably have to have some deconditioning dialogues with your addiction-memory:

ADDICTED BRAIN: "Beer . . . that just calls for a cigarette."
NONSMOKING BRAIN TO ADDICTED BRAIN: "Oh, back to Pavlov. Hello, addicted 'upstairs'; didn't you get it? Automated smoking with alcohol is done for. Licking an ashtray does not improve the taste of beer. Plus, I can have fun without it. No discussion."
ADDICTED BRAIN: "Well, but the old times were so nice . . . are you sure you don't want one?"
NONSMOKING BRAIN: "Forget it! I am not going to fall for that anymore. Damn the old smoke stress and loss of freedom. I'm done listening to you."

ADDICTED BRAIN: "Now, if you'd have a little cigarette with your coffee, you might enjoy it more."
NONSMOKING BRAIN TO CONDITIONED BRAIN: "I have purchased an expensive, good espresso brand and I will not ruin the flavor with tar, smoke, and chemicals."
ADDICTED BRAIN: "But you've always . . ."
NONSMOKING BRAIN: "'Always' was yesterday. I am no longer on autopilot, and by the way, I like being able to actually taste things again."

ADDICTED BRAIN: "Why don't you smoke one . . . it's just part of being at the pub."
NONSMOKING BRAIN TO ADDICTED BRAIN: "Oh, yes, so I'll have to run outside every half an hour. And tomorrow morning I'll be coughing and will smell of smoke. Give it up. Pub

and cigarettes don't go together at all. Unless you want to stand alone outside."

ADDICTED BRAIN: "But . . ."

NONSMOKING BRAIN: "No buts; discussion closed."

ADDICTED BRAIN: "This boredom while waiting . . . why don't you light one?"

NONSMOKING BRAIN TO ADDICTED BRAIN: "Smoking does not make waiting more pleasant. Now stop your whining."

ADDICTED BRAIN: "There's just so much stress today! Come on, smoke—it'll relax you."

NONSMOKING BRAIN TO ADDICTED BRAIN: "That's what I tried for years, and I know I'll be even *more* stressed in half an hour from the nicotine."

ADDICTED BRAIN: "But for that half hour you will feel good."

NONSMOKING BRAIN: "Very funny, but I'm tired of that emotional roller coaster."

THE BOTTOM LINE

- ▶ The drug nicotine conditions everyday situations into smoking triggers. The feeling that you are smoking "just like that" and "always when . . ." are typical for these triggered cigarettes.
- ▶ The conditioned smoking behavior is stored in the same part of the brain as that of survival behaviors. Therefore, it can lead to panic when you are not allowed to smoke.
- ▶ It takes several weeks to unlearn these conditioned smoking cues, but then they are completely gone and don't cause any further desire to smoke.
- ▶ You need a bit of humor to step back and retrain your brain.

12

Your Cigarette Brand and Other Smokers

Why Do Smokers Have Such High Brand Loyalty?

Lovingly we stroke our packs of cigarettes, until we may smoke at last. Yes, we love our brand. It has always amazed marketing strategists: Smokers have a brand loyalty that is hard to explain, by far the highest brand loyalty of all consumer goods. If pressed, smokers will switch brands for health reasons, such as from Marlboro to a lighter Marlboro. However, in blind tests, smokers can rarely pick their cigarette brand. Despite this, smokers always declare they are "extremely satisfied" with their product. The desired effect, to eliminate the nicotine withdrawal symptoms, is immediate from hit to hit.

Habits and preferences, however, ordinarily change frequently. For example, if you have bought vanilla yogurt for 6 months and you are then tired of vanilla, you switch to a different flavor. This is precisely where the difference lies between well-conditioned "addiction consumer products" and vanilla yogurt. As a teenager, you probably identified yourself with a brand that had a particular image. But now that you are a permanent smoker—likely still smoking that same brand—do you even notice cigarette advertising? Probably not. The world of brands soon hides behind the addiction. The high level of brand loyalty of adult smokers can be explained only by the special conditioning of the particular cigarette brand. Let's take Marlboro. With each Marlboro cigarette, the neurotransmitter dopamine in the brain is released. This activates, amplifies, and reinforces memorizing, remembering, and learning. You learn what temporarily "feels good," store it in your brain, and associate this with the small pack in your hand. So you connect many alleviating moments with your Marlboro cigarette. A life without cigarettes, and without *that specific brand of cigarettes*, becomes hard to imagine. This is deeply learned and stored in the brain. Advertising for a different brand is not very effective compared to intensive conditioning with "your" cigarettes. Too many times smoking your brand of cigarettes has gotten you out of an unsatisfactory, uneasy mood and given you short-term relief. At 20 cigarettes a day, this comes to 73,000 temporarily relaxing Marlboro moments in 10 years. No vanilla yogurt could ever produce such brand loyalty. Nicotine addiction is a customer loyalty program, and conditioned learning ensures that you are the most loyal brand junkie of any consumer product.

Other Smokers

Are smokers nicer people? We all love those smoking corners. It is much easier to connect than anywhere else. Smokers sympathize with one another and are more accessible. This is at least how smokers like to see themselves. When someone asks for a cigarette, most smokers will respond positively and generally help out. Do they do this because they are nicer than nonsmokers? Can you look at it like that? After all, a nonsmoker can rarely give such joy if you want to smoke *now*. Does that not prove it? These people must be nicer. But do smokers help out of sympathy? Probably not. Everyone who smokes knows exactly the nervous, unbearable feeling when you *need* a cigarette *right now*. There is an unspoken code of conduct among smokers to help out when another smoker has a craving or feels withdrawal, because every smoker knows how bad this feels and that it could happen to them as well. Advertising reinterprets this "withdrawal assistance" as communicative, open, and generous: a friendly, smiling smoker offering a cigarette to a complete stranger. In reality, most of us would prefer to immerse ourselves in conversations with scroungers as little as possible. Unless it is a particularly attractive woman or man. But how often does this really happen? Most smokers simply smoke to eliminate their addiction and happen to be standing next to each other. Think about it: How many times do you stand next to another and just smoke in silence? You aren´t smoking for companionship; you just happen to need your nicotine at the same time.

THE BOTTOM LINE

- ▶ See cigarettes for what they really are: a banal, well-conditioned addictive product that fills the coffers of nicotine dealers.
- ▶ Other smokers are not friendlier people, just fellow addicts with whom you often just happen to smoke to eliminate your own feelings of withdrawal.

 BRAVO! You have earned the second star. You have read 2 parts of this book. You have already come very, very far.

Part 3

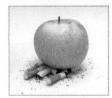

Other Reasons to Quit Smoking

13

Weight and Beauty

Smoking Neither Makes You Beautiful Nor Keeps You Slim

"If I stop smoking I will put on weight." It is women, in particular, who use this fear of putting on the extra pounds as the perfect excuse for not quitting smoking. This is understandable. All people—male and female—want to look attractive, receive attention, and like what they see when they look in the mirror. It's simply a good feeling. An acceptable body, your self-image, your sexy flirt factor, and the way you feel in general—these are all interdependent. But lingering over reflection from only a yard or 2 away focuses the vision far too much on body shape. The classic situation: A woman standing in front of the mirror moves around constantly, examining herself from all angles, until she finds something wrong with herself. How does a guy view himself in the mirror? He stands right in front of it, motionless, for a short period of time. Then all is good. "I look okay," the guy thinks. End of story. Hardly any guy would keep turning and looking at himself from unfortunate angles, seeking dissatisfaction with whatever he is seeing.

Using a mirror to judge the attractiveness of your body is a fatal mistake. Being attractive involves a lot more than simply having a good body. It includes having nice white teeth; a good complexion and smooth, pleasant-smelling skin; no bad breath; shiny, thick hair, clear, healthy eyes; a clear speaking voice, being able to laugh without needing to clear the throat first . . . an all-around image of fitness and a relaxed stress-free mood. That's sexy! But all of these personal characteristics are simply ruined by cigarettes. The toxic substances make your hair become thinner and turn gray prematurely, your skin become pale and age faster, the whites of your eyes take on a yellowish cast, and your stained teeth look anything but good. Bad breath and a general, unpleasant body odor kill any eroticism. A hoarse voice sounds as if you have a cold and doesn't add to your overall appeal. On top of this, a certain "bitchiness" kicks in when your nicotine level drops too quickly—that's not the recipe for being attractive. But you don't see that in your mirrored body image. Attractiveness is much more than having a great body. Quitting smoking will help you get it all back again.

The Big Sexy Flirt Test

When did you last think about how you flirt? 69% of men and 72% of women are nonsmokers. For this group, smoking is anything but cool, and by no stretch of the imagination is it sexy or sophisticated. It is simply accepted or tolerated because people like you anyway. You are liked *in spite of* and not *because of* your smoking. So, take the big partner/flirt factor test. As you do, keep in mind that smokers on average *temporarily* gain about 6 pounds when they quit smoking.[72]

Mark an X next to what you believe a bit more weight after quitting really means.

❏ True ❏ False: It's better to flirt with someone who weighs on additional 6 pounds than with someone whose mouth and lungs smell of tar, whose hair has a stale smell, and whose skin exudes smoke from every pore.

❏ True ❏ False: It's more attractive to kiss someone who weighs 6 pounds more than someone with whom you have the feeling of licking an ashtray.

❏ True ❏ False: I would rather be with someone who weighs an additional 6 pounds for a short time than with someone who always has pallid skin and yellow teeth.

❏ True ❏ False: I would prefer someone who temporarily has an additional 6 pounds' weight to someone whose skin has aged by 10 years and simply looks old.

❏ True ❏ False: Someone who weighs 6 pounds more for a couple of months is more appealing than someone with a permanent cough, who hacks up phlegm, and has a hoarse, smoky voice.

❏ True ❏ False: I would prefer someone with 6 pounds' more weight than someone who is sickly and who may die 8 years earlier.

❏ True ❏ False: It is better to be with someone who weighs an additional 6 pounds for a short time but who, on the other hand, is more active and fit to do lots of things.

❏ True ❏ False: I would rather be with someone who temporarily has 6 pounds' more weight than to be with someone who constantly deprives me of clean air in my own home.

❏ True ❏ False: It is better to flirt with someone who weighs an additional 6 pounds than with someone who constantly has to disappear for a cigarette during a romantic meal or else is unbearably nervous.

How Attractive Are You Really?

How did you do on the test? Ouch—that was predictable and biased, right? The fact remains, however, that smoking is not attractive . . . or do you disagree? Your figure is only a small part of what makes up your attractiveness. Genuine smokers like to see themselves as sophisticated, fascinating, and sexy. This self-image has been placed in the heads of smokers by the million-dollar campaigns funded by the tobacco industry. However, nonsmokers don't fall for this. They trust their instinct when they sniff a smoker or inhale clouds of toxic substances. Don't just take my word for it. The test you just took is the result of a nationwide survey in Germany,[73] which revealed that only 8% of nonsmokers find smokers sexy. 14% refused to date smokers! 12% said they would never have sex with a smoker! More than 50% found their partner's smoking habits disgusting. And what about the self-image of the smoker? Only 6% of smokers believed that smoking was the reason why they were refused a date. The self-image and other people's image of a smoker just don't correspond.

Not smoking improves your skin and your breath, you age more slowly, you smell better, and you are no longer at the mercy of addiction. Overall, you become more attractive for many people. The advantages far outweigh the chance that you *might temporarily* put on a few pounds. You can rid yourself of this extra weight soon and I am going to show you how to even avoid putting it on in the first place.

Then factor in the health risks of smoking that you've known for ages. "I won't stop smoking because I'll put on weight," is really one of the most flimsy excuses to continue inhaling nicotine, one that is whispered to you directly from your addicted brain. If you have a sticky note handy, write this on it and stick it to your mirror, "I would rather be sexy and attractive than a smoker."

It is a myth that smoking keeps you thin. More on why smokers are no slimmer than nonsmokers and how you can keep your weight in check when you quit can be found in part 4 of this book. But for now, please continue reading about the other physical benefits of quitting.

Not Smoking Is the Best Antiaging Treatment

It is a fact that smokers age significantly faster than nonsmokers do. What would your skin look like if you didn't smoke? You can find out more about this taking the example of pictures of twins where one smokes and the other one doesn't. Slower aging, smelling better, and becoming more attractive motivates many to quit smoking. Work on Day 7 of the Internet program to get a strong motivation for quitting.

DAY 7
of the Internet program

THE BOTTOM LINE

- ▶ Smokers imagine themselves more attractive than others view them in reality.
- ▶ Cigarettes neither keep you slim nor make you sexy.
- ▶ Smokers are not slimmer than nonsmokers.
- ▶ Smoking makes the body age faster and ruins hair, teeth, and skin.
- ▶ Quitting makes you more attractive and appealing.

14

The Daily Cocktail of Chemicals

I COULD ABSOLUTELY IGNORE THE LITTLE bit of tar (elegantly termed condensate) and carbon monoxide shown on the side of a pack. I knew like all smokers that cigarettes contain toxic substances. But I really didn't want to know, in all their glorious details, what I was really inhaling. Although, when I finally looked into things, it really did help to know, as a reason to resolve to quit.

Please—before you slam the book closed because you don't want to get into the particulars of this ugly truth, read on a little. Light up a cigarette. You'll have finished the chapter by the time you've finished it.

Tobacco smoke is a complex chemical mixture containing up to 4,800 combustion products,[74] 2,000 of which are known to be toxic substances. With the 600 additives from the tobacco industry alone, you're gassing yourself with a chemical mixture that is difficult to analyze.

"Difficult to analyze" doesn't mean they do not affect your

body. There is an abundance of evidence that smoking causes cancer: fully 90 individual substances in tobacco smoke have been classified as carcinogenic.[75] No minimum ("safe") level can be set for carcinogenic substances for when they do not cause damage. Even the smallest amounts of these substances can cause cells to degenerate.

Day after day, smokers inhale a poisonous cocktail of dioxin, nitrosamines, heavy metals, benzenes, polycyclic hydrocarbons, arsenic, cadmium, formaldehyde . . . the list goes on and on. Both "lights" and "ultra lights," introduced in the 1990s, contain exactly the same amount of toxic and carcinogenic substances in the tobacco smoked. Cigarettes containing no additives are no better. New advertising slogans, devised to make cigarettes without additives look healthier, deliberately confuse the smoker with the suggestion that smoking such products is actually healthy, so as to keep them smoking. Naturally, these stultifying advertisements appear just before the end of the year to stop smokers from resolving to quit.

"I Just Smoke for the Pleasure of It"

Once inhaled, the highly toxic particles and gases form a fine poisonous film on the mucous membranes in the mouth, throat, and lungs. The alveoli (air sacs) in the lungs have a total surface of some 1,500 yards square—the size of a tennis court. Even the most fleeting of highly toxic gaseous substances dissolve in the moisture film of the lungs' alveoli and from there are transported throughout your body. Anyone can see immediately that this is anything but good for you.

The consequences of these cancerous cocktails: 92% of all cancers of the mouth, 90% of all lung cancer cases, 81% of all cancers of the larynx, and 78% of all cancers of the esophagus in men are directly attributable to smoking. Cancer incidence in many other organs increases dramatically as these carcinogenic substances are transported further throughout the body. 30% of all cancer cases in the EU are caused by smoking. One reason: The toxic substances activate cancer genes that otherwise wouldn't be decoded (read) from your genetic software. These toxins also change and block certain repair genes even years after quitting.[76]

So, when you say, "I smoke just for the pleasure of it," what a morbid pleasure it is: inhaling day after day a carcinogenic toxic film settling on your mucous membranes. 1 smoker in 2 pays for this "pleasure" with his or her life at a much too early age—5 million people throughout the world annually.

"But Pollution Is Just as Bad"

Cigarettes exceed any permitted limit for environmental pollution by far. Smoking just 20 cigarettes daily means you are personally exceeding, within your immediate environment, the particulate air pollution limits in Germany by a thousandfold. And let's go back to the 90 carcinogenic substances specific to cigarettes. Here is a small selection of what they are.[77] The data is in milligrams (mg), micrograms (mcg), or nanograms (ng). Enjoy!

Acetaldehyde 980 mcg–1.37 mg, acrylonitrile 1–2 mg, 4-aminobiphenyl 0.2–23 ng, o-anisidine hydrochloride, arsenic, benzene 5.9–75 mcg, beryllium 0.5 ng, 1.3-butadiene 152–400 mcg, cadmium 1.7 mcg, 1.1-dimethylhydrazine, ethylene oxide, formaldehyde, furan, heterocyclic amines, hydrazine 32 mcg, isoprene 3.1 mg, lead 2-naphthylamine 1.5–35 ng, nitromethane n-nitrosodi-n-butylamine 3 ng, n-nitrosodiethanolamine 24-36 ng, n-nitrosodiethylamine up to 8.3 ng, n-nitrosodimethylamine 5.7–43 ng, n-nitrosodi-n-propylamine 1 ng, 4-(n-nitrosomethylamino)-1-(3-pyridyl)-1-butanone 4.2

mcg, n-nitrosonornicotine 14 mcg, n-nitrosopiperidine n-nitroso-pyrrolidine 113 ng, n-nitrososarcosine 22–460 ng, polonium-210, polycyclic aromatic hydrocarbons 28–100 mg, o-toluidine 32 ng, vinyl chloride 5.6–27 ng

This list doesn't even contain the additional 4,800 molecules contained in smoke, which have never been tested as to their health effects.

So why am I giving you this list? It confronts you with the real facts: It's not just a matter of a little tar or carbon monoxide, which is printed on the side of the pack. If you gas yourself for years with dozens of carcinogenic substances, it is obvious that your genetic makeup is being affected by the toxins you are breathing. Long before someone is diagnosed with cancer as a result of smoking, changes can be found in the cells in the mouth, throat, lungs, and bladder. These are known as precancerous cells. The good news is: Many of these precancerous cells regress when you quit smoking. When you quit early enough. So set a quitting date before it is too late.

A Brief Word to Pregnant Women: Your Fetus Is Smoking Along with You

The thousands of toxic substances in tobacco smoke reach the bloodstream of your unborn child through the umbilical cord. Your fetus is defenseless against them. Carcinogenic substances, such as polycyclic aromatic hydrocarbons and tobacco-specific nitrosamines, can cause damage to the genes of a developing fetus, and often results in the birth of deformed children.[78] Other substances, such as lead, hinder the development of a baby's brain. A small, unborn child is in a much less capable position of coping with these toxic substances in comparison to the adult body, as the organs required to do so are insufficiently developed. Moreover, the high number of poisonous substances produced by tobacco increases the risk of miscarriage and still-birth by 30% and leads to twice the frequency of premature births in female smokers.[79] Shortly before giving birth, 20% of pregnant women smoke on average 13 cigarettes per day. This amounts to 3,640 cigarettes in 9 months, or 36,400 poisonous inhalations. Smoking during pregnancy is a form of child abuse.

Switch Off Your Own Nuclear Power Station!

Surely you watched spellbound as the worst-case nuclear scenario at Fukushima and thought about the unfolded health consequences caused by radioactive contamination. We still remember with horror when the radioactive clouds of Chernobyl turned in the wrong direction. The heroes of Chernobyl and Fukushima had either no or inadequate protective clothing. But they always had one thing: respiratory protection so that the radioactive particles could not reach the alveoli in their lungs. This is in stark contrast to smokers.

The tobacco plant does an excellent job of accumulating polonium-210 and lead-210. These are released in the combustion process and 10% is contained in the smoke you inhale. Both radioactive particles are found in the exterior lung tissue of smokers. In the case of smokers, this radioactivity has been measured as up to 100 times greater than in the rest of the lung. Tobacco can be up to 1,000 times more radioactive than the leaves of trees found directly adjacent to Chernobyl. Polonium-210 radiates 1,000 times stronger than plutonium or caesium-123, which rained down upon us from Chernobyl and on Japan!

Directly and daily, as long as you continue to smoke, you inhale polonium-210 and lead-210 right into your lungs where the dangerous alpha rays have a particularly strong effect.

Cigarettes are your personal mini nuclear plant, right inside your mouth.

Radiating Beautifully Through Smoking

Are you glowing yet? The yearly radiation dose of someone who smokes 20 cigarettes per day is equal to some 250 X-rays of the lung.[80] Or to put it more technically, 106 millisieverts (mSv) of radiation are reached annually by smoking 20 cigarettes daily. To put this in perspective,[81] 10 mSv—less than one tenth of that amount—is the maximum annual dose for workers in Australian uranium mines. Employees in nuclear power plants and other professions where they are exposed to radiation are permitted an annual maximum dosage of no greater than 20 mSv for the entire body. That is the highest permissible dosage! Yet smokers consuming a pack per day are exposed to 5 times this maximum limit. And smokers annually absorb 100 times the level of radiation considered safe for the resident population near a nuclear plant.

Cancer incidence increases above 100 mSv of annual exposure, according to the World Nuclear Association; 350 mSv per year of constant radiation at home was the official criterion for resettling the population in Fukushima and Chernobyl after the nuclear accidents. Do you smoke some 40 cigarettes daily? Then you are exposing yourself regularly to 206 millisieverts annually over the next 20 years. That should make you radiate beautifully. Inhalation of radioactive particles is dangerous for the alveoli in the lungs. Only recently has it been discovered that constant exposure to radiation causes more than half of the cancer cases in smokers. Radioactive pollonium-210 and lead-210, in particular, are the greatest health risks affecting the tobacco industry. Cigarette packs should have had a radioactive warning on them a long time ago, and the amount of radioactive substances should be listed. This should be in place of those belittling tar warnings that must be printed on the packs. That alone should tell you something: Both the cigarette and the nuclear energy industries have something in common when it comes to risks. Risks are concealed, data falsified and minimized. Information is withheld from smokers, just like after a nuclear incident.

Additives to Increase Acceptance

For some years you have had to smoke new additives designed to make cigarettes more socially acceptable. One of the major marketing challenges for the industry was the recent evolution of militant antismokers who felt bothered by smoke and fought to ban smoking. As a result the tobacco industry has been researching frantically over the past 20 years to see how, through additives, it could reduce the visibility of smoke, reduce the irritation it causes, and improve its smell. The less visible and annoying the smoke would be, they thought, the fewer nonsmokers would complain.

The companies' interest was not to reduce the thousands of toxic and damaging substances in cigarettes. You could guess that the industry is really not all that concerned about the health of nonsmokers . . . the goal is to use even *more* chemicals to reduce the visibility and stench of smoke, and thus to ensure that smokers keep right on smoking.

There are some 300 industry patents for these additives alone.[82] Whether these new chemical molecules that develop in the combustion of additives are additionally toxic was hardly tested by any independent scientists. Smokers now inhale more chemicals to increase social acceptance. Smokers are extremely considerate individuals! And all of this only to ensure the profits of the nicotine industry. These additives include:

- **FOR A BETTER AROMA:** acetylpyrazine, anethole, beta-caryophyllene, cedrol, ethyl 3-methylvalerate, furaneol, limonene, p-anisaldehyde, phenethyl alcohol, "Aromatek 150," "Aromatek 245"
- **FOR LESS IRRITATION:** aluminium sulfate, (NH4)2So4, NaH2Po4, "XLF-636," "XLF-662," "XLF-680," "XLF-755"
- **FOR LESS VISIBILITY:** alumina sol-gel, MgCo3 sol-gel, MgCo3, H3Po4, K2P2O7, CaCo3, calcium carbonate, Na2Co3 (sodium carbonate), calcium chloride, citric acid, magnesium oxide, potassium acetate, potassium citrate, sodium hexametaphosphate, glutaric acid, hydromagnesite, malonic acid, potassium phosphate, magnesite, potassium succinate, magnesium carbonate, monobasic potassium phosphate, calcium carbonate, monopotassium phosphate, "Studio 26 blend," "XTH Studio blend"

Get Out of Breath Faster and Have Less Concentration

When you smoke, carbon monoxide will occupy your red blood cells instead of oxygen. Carbon monoxide bonds 300 times better to red blood cells than oxygen does. This prevents oxygen from reaching the red blood cells. That is to say, all the areas of a smoker's body are receiving insufficient oxygen, blocked by the repeated influx of carbon monoxide. And this is exactly when you start gasping for air. It can take 6 hours without a cigarette for the carbon monoxide to begin to break down and leave room for more oxygen in the blood cells.

Carbon monoxide is a highly poisonous, odorless gas. It causes most people to get dizzy and feel sick after their very first cigarette. Those who smoke only now and again experience this dizziness constantly. So why do smokers who smoke daily never feel dizzy? Smokers produce more red blood cells so that the cells get oxygen somehow. This improves the supply of oxygen but makes the blood thicker and can lead to small blood vessels' getting blocked.

I am sure you have often had headaches after having smoked away the evening. No wonder. Headaches, a slight feeling of nausea, and dizziness are the typical symptoms of mild carbon monoxide poisoning when too little oxygen is supplied to the body. Smokers feel as if a cold is coming on. Even the following morning, they may have a hangover from oxygen deprivation and cough up dirt out of their lungs. This is the very best time to quit smoking. No one hates smoking more than on such a morning.

Have you ever asked yourself why race car drivers don't smoke? Even though some teams accept the money and wear Marlboro suits they never risk smoking. The lack of oxygen would have made them unconcentrated and tired. Although nicotine in and of itself increases concentration somewhat, that "positive" effect is completely destroyed by the very act of smoking, which overloads your red blood cells with carbon monoxide. Oxygen deprivation leads to wooziness, not focus. So, smoking cigarettes in no way helps you concentrate better. If you have the feeling that you can concentrate better after a cigarette, this is usually because your withdrawal symptoms, such as restlessness and nervousness, have been temporarily reduced by your getting a new dose of nicotine. But that "improvement" is just the selective and subjective perception of the smoker. In the case of more complex and creative mental tasks, time and again, studies have shown smokers perform worse.

A Brief Word for Pregnant Women: Carbon Monoxide and Nicotine

Carbon monoxide reduces the supply of oxygen to the unborn child if the mother smokes during pregnancy. In addition, nicotine narrows blood vessels, including those to the placenta. Thus, the fetus receives less oxygen. This is like turning off the oxygen supply to a diver who is under water. The baby's heart functions are impaired. In addition, oxygen deprivation can lead to growth and developmental disorders, not only in the brain, affecting not only intelligence, but potentially damaging other organs. Many miscarriages, premature babies, and stillbirths are the consequence of carbon monoxide in the mother's bloodstream. Even following a successful delivery, this early oxygen deprivation continues to negatively affect the child's health: Sudden infant death syndrome—the third most common cause of death for babies—can be reduced by half if the mother doesn't smoke during pregnancy.

Many pregnant women would love to stop smoking if they only knew how. Mothers-to-be are also very successful in quitting: 10 times as many pregnant women manage to quit smoking in comparison to other smokers trying to quit.[83] Why not be one of them? In spite of this success rate in the United States, still one tenth of all pregnant women turn off the oxygen supply to the unborn child several times a day just weeks before giving birth. It is never too soon to stop smoking if you are pregnant.

"Oh, Leave Me Alone, I Inhale More Carbon Monoxide on a Busy Road."

Whether you smoke a cigarette or put your face directly in front of the exhaust pipe of a car, you get about the same amount of carbon monoxide. Smokers inhale about 1,000 times more than is permitted as the maximum at the workplace.[84]

Here is a comparison of carbon monoxide concentrations:

fresh sea air	0.06 ppm
maximum concentration at the workplace	30 ppm
street corner	5–50 ppm
heavy traffic	50–100 ppm
cigarette smoke	20,000–60,000 ppm
inhaling directly from a car exhaust	30,000–80,000 ppm

"It Doesn't Matter. I Don't Feel Any Damage."

You just haven't really noticed it . . . yet. But carbon monoxide is particularly active on your arterial walls. Through a variety of inflammatory processes, it causes more fat to be deposited there. You are as young and healthy as your blood vessels. The blood vessels of smokers who have smoked for a lifetime are full of deposited fat, which leads to the blockage of blood vessels going to the heart, the brain, the kidneys, and also the feet. The risk of a stroke or heart attack increases and smokers' legs often have to be amputated. When male smokers need good blood vessels that expand and give volume, these are commonly blocked or do not receive sufficient blood. Impotence is usually the result. Carbon monoxide definitely has long-term effects even if you are not feeling them yet.

"Of Course That Doesn't Affect Me. Something's Got to Kill You."

This is the ultimate defense of a smoker. It shows how uninformed he is. Or the smoker has come to terms with the fact that he still doesn´t know how to break out of the deadly smokers' prison.

Imagine the scandal if 4,800 toxic substances were found in chocolate. The television stations would be flooded with news specials, government spokesmen would make statements, and the guilty would be found even in politics. Heads would roll. There would be calls for the immediate withdrawal of approval to market chocolate. With 140,000 deaths from chocolate in Germany alone, the CEOs of the chocolate companies there would be up for manslaughter. The only difference from tobacco is that there is no chocolate tax, the former making up the fourth-largest revenue in the state budget, at least in Germany as well as significantly in many other countries.

The decision is yours. Would you let the toss of a coin decide your life? Half of smokers die prematurely, because they smoke. Smokers die on average 10 years younger than nonsmokers do. If you smoke to the end of your life without having had breaks, then on average you die even 14 years younger. Only 59% of smokers reach the age of 70. And no wonder, when you think of all the highly poisonous substances passing from each cigarette into their lungs. If smoking 20 cigarettes per day, that amounts to some 73,000 toxic inhalations per year, multiply that by 20 years and that is 1.4 million toxic inhalations, which will have caused major changes to a body's cells.

The fear for your life is a very real one. But the fear that you will never enjoy life as much again without a cigarette is purely a figment of your imagination. It feels real but will last only as long as you smoke and are dependent on nicotine. In 2009, an estimated 46.6 million, or 20.6% of American adults (aged 18+) were current smokers. The number of smokers declined 50% between 1965 and 2009. All of these ex-smokers seem to be missing nothing. Otherwise you would hear constant moaning and how much they would long to continue smoking.

Look Toward the Future

"Oh, now I really feel awful that for years I've been doing this to my body." Forget that immediately. Blaming yourself never helps. Addiction makes everyone do some crazy things. The only important thing is to look toward the future. Make the decision to stop using your body as a dumping ground for toxic waste. Without this stress you'll soon feel a lot better.

THE BOTTOM LINE

- ► As long as you smoke, you inhale a chemical cocktail of 4,800 toxic particles from combustion, 90 carcinogenic substances, and 600 nondeclared additives daily.
- ► The carbon monoxide and fine particle intake of a smoker is 1,000 times higher than permitted levels.
- ► The radioactive levels of a smoker are 5 times that of the maximum allowed exposure in a nuclear power plant.
- ► Smoking 20 cigarettes daily, or 73,000 chemical and radioactive poisonous inhalations annually, cannot help but negatively affect on your health.

15

The Dewy-Eyed View of Risks

IT'S GREAT THAT YOU'RE STILL HERE and reading away. Just so you know in advance, we are now getting down to business: Let's take a look together at the 6 most common tricks that smokers use to circumvent all the obstacles and continue smoking. Smokers distort their own perception of health risks with a mixture of mysterious individual excuses and naive thoughts that are far removed from reality. This self-constructed perception of risk is completely different from the real risks. Of course every smoker knows this. Here are the most common means of self-deception.

Strategy 1: Remaining Naive

"If smoking is really so damaging, then cigarettes would have been banned years ago." If cigarettes were a consumer product like any other, as the cigarette industry maintains it is, why does it kill more than 440,000 Americans each year and cost more than $96 billion in medical costs? Many smokers use the "naive strategy" to refute these numbers and responsibility is passed on to the higher authority. Strangely enough, though, the same argument (then cigarettes would have been banned years ago) is used by the lobby organizations of the cigarette industry.[85]

But you are responsible for your own actions. The reality is: 5 million smokers die globally every year as a result of smoking. The average smoker's life expectancy is reduced by 10 years.

"Oh, how can you be so sure of the facts?" From studies of survivors. Let us take, for example, 34,000 British doctors who collected death and disease data over a period of 50 years.[86] And to avoid from the outset getting into a fight over details as to whether smoking causes this or that type of cancer, the end result that counted was simply survival time. This was considerably longer in subjects who did not smoke. Imagine your best 10 friends smoking and imagine how many of them will still be alive at the age of 60, 70, or 80.

93% of nonsmokers are still alive at 60,

but only 79% of smokers.

85% of nonsmokers are still alive at 70,

but only 57% of smokers.

59% of nonsmokers are still alive at 80,

but only 26% of smokers.

Strategy 2: Belittling or Comparing the Risks

"Whether I smoke or not, there is always a risk somewhere. I could die in a plane crash." Okay, but would you get into an aircraft if every fifth one crashed? The worse a risk appears and the less influence you have over it, the higher the risk seems. Terrorist attacks, airplane disasters, tsunamis are all seen as threats. The probability of their happening is minimal. This is not the case with the risks of smoking. The probability of their happening is extremely high for smokers.

🚶🚶🧍🧍🧍🧍🧍🧍🧍🧍 20% of all deaths in men over age 35 are solely attributable to smoking.[87]

"Nah; environmental pollution, such as exhaust fumes, is just as bad for your health." Every year, if you are a smoker, your lungs get a cupful of tar and the amount of fine dust particles that you take in is 1,000 times above the maximum limit. This first makes itself apparent though a lack of breath and a smoker's cough, and ends with almost total loss of function of the lungs, known as COPD (chronic obstructive pulmonary disease). The lung tissue in those who have COPD can scarcely absorb oxygen. You basically suffocate. Many smokers haven't even heard of COPD although it is the third most common cause of death among smokers. Of the 20,710 German COPD deaths in 2006, 90% were smokers. (You can read more about COPD in the Internet learning program, Day 8.)

🧍🧍🧍🧍🧍🧍🧍🧍🧍🧍 90% of COPD sufferers are smokers.

Strategy 3: Seemingly Controlling the Risks

Risks that one believes one can influence or that one takes voluntarily are judged to be controllable.

"Yes, I smoke but I eat healthy." You cannot control the 4,800 toxins or the 90 carcinogens in smoke, or counterbalance them with organically grown fruit. It is simply a fallacy. Some 30% of all cancer cases are attributable to smoking alone. Some forms of cancer appear in far greater proportion among smokers than in nonsmokers, as you can see in the figures below.[88] Let us take the example of lung cancer: in Germany, 42,000 men and women die from it every year. That is equal to 120 jumbo jets crashing annually—one completely filled jumbo jet every 3 days. Madness. Lung cancer is the fourth most common cause of death.

The casualties of actual air disasters, earthquakes, or terrorist attacks are inflated by the media. But smokers crash every day. Quietly. Without reports in the media. Globally, some 1.2 million smokers, or 3,428 jumbo jets' worth of passengers, die unnecessarily every year because of their addiction to tobacco. You can see how distorted the risk perception of smokers and the media really is. As long as you smoke, you are in control of nothing.

Proportion of smokers in cases of lung cancer: 90%

Proportion of smokers in cases of mouth cancer: 92%

Proportion of smokers in cases of cancer of the larynx: 81%

Proportion of smokers in cases of cancer of the esophagus: 78%

50% of all kidney and bladder cancers in men are attributable to smoking.[89]

"That is why I smoke lights or cigarettes without additives." This is absolute nonsense: you do not avoid the carcinogenic substances.

"I smoke of my own accord." A risk is no smaller because you take it voluntarily.

"I will stop early enough." Risks, which will occur in 10 to 20 years, seem smaller, although the probability is higher. When is early enough, exactly? Degenerated cells in the lungs can be found early on in smokers.

"You have to die anyway. Cigarettes speed things up just a bit." The latter is true, as you can see below—but do you truly wish to die before your time?

23% of cancer cases in women are diagnosed under the age of 50.[90]

90% of all heart attacks in people under age 40 are smokers.

Half of all deaths caused by smoking tobacco occur between the ages of 35 and 69. Paying into pension plans is unnecessary for half of all smokers. They will never live to see their pensions.

Strategy 4: Denying the Risks

"I don't believe any of it. I am not interested in what is printed on the pack." Denial does not reduce the real risks. Many smokers despise themselves because of this—they know that they are smoking themselves to death because of addiction.

"So what? I am sure whether you get sick or not depends on your personal constitution. I've been smoking for 20 years and I'm as fit as a fiddle." Okay. Let us take a look at what smoking does when people's genetic material is exactly the same. How? By examining the cause of death of 1,515 twins born between 1917 and 1929. One of each pair of twins smoked and the other didn't. This shows the results with people having the same genetic makeup. The risk of death before reaching the age of 60 doubled in smokers. In the case of heavy smokers, the risk tripled. In addition, the risk of death from cardiovascular diseases was 4 times higher; of dying from cancer, 3 times higher; and in the case of lung cancer, 5 times higher. The risk is not reduced because you overestimate your physical constitution and your health. In particular, men and younger people tend toward such fantasies of being invulnerable.

"Hey, I could die in a traffic accident." It is amazing how smokers equip their cars: safety belts, ABS, airbags. Who would want to crash and die 10 years early? In Germany, 4,050 people died in car accidents in 2009. In that same year, only half that number died of esophageal, mouth, or throat cancer (1,856 cases), and 4 times as many suffocated from COPD (20,710 cases). 10 times as many died of lung cancer (42,000 cases). All these diseases appear almost exclusively in smokers. A further 30% were attributable to the increased risk of strokes or heart attacks. There were 34 times more deaths caused by smoking than by traffic accidents in just that one year, 2009. "But you have to die of something and that doesn't apply to me," does not really work.

Deaths in Thousands for Germany

👤👤👤👤 4,050 deaths in traffic accidents

👤👤 1,856 deaths from mouth, esophageal and throat cancer (92% of whom were smokers)

👤👤👤👤👤👤👤👤👤👤👤👤👤👤👤👤👤👤👤👤👤👤👤 20,710 deaths from COPD (90% of whom were smokers)

👤👤 42,000 deaths from lung cancer (85% of whom were smokers)

A total of 140,000 people died as a direct result of smoking.

Strategy 5: Reacting as If You Are Overwhelmed

"I don't know what to believe. This all doesn't seem to be based on proven facts. I'll just continue smoking." The cigarette industry has been banking on this for years. Its classic strategy is to hide the truth for as long as possible, deny the risks, and pay for research to suit the industry's ends, confusing the smoker with biased figures. As a result, reputable academic journals no longer accept research articles if they are sponsored by the tobacco industry. All too often these were manipulated. The worst strategy is to believe nicotine dealers.

If the numbers presented in this chapter's figures seem overwhelming, keep your eye on the 4,800 toxic substances that cause damage and countless lethal diseases throughout the body. That number is an indisputable fact.

Strategy 6: Justifying Your Actions—Balancing the Risks and Benefits

"You have to die of something and I'm enjoying life *now*." With some benefits, risks are more readily accepted. But smoking has no advantages for the mind. It makes you more prone to stress, more restless, and more irritable. The health risks cannot be offset by adding the supposed benefits of smoking into a twisted calculation. This is the most frequent justification smokers believe in.

The well-worn excuse "You have to die of something" is just as strange. Unfortunately, you don´t die quickly. On average, when nonsmoking seniors self-rate their health, they say they spent 68 years in "good health." Smokers self-rate their health as "good health" on average only up to the age of 56.[91] They don't even reach a seniority of healthy years. That means you lose one decade in which you no longer feel healthy and fit before finally dying 10 to 14 years prematurely. The "I'm enjoying life *now*" argument just doesn´t sound so good anymore. The resulting promise is not enjoyment, but slow death. Get real. Quit now.

"Smoking Kills in 24 Different Ways."

I find this sentence memorable. It is an introduction to a study by the European Union,[92] which lists the directly proven killer diseases caused by tobacco consumption: COPD, heart attack, stroke, and a dozen types of different cancers. Your health provides great motivation for quitting. Give those cigarettes one last kick with Day 8 of the internet program

 DAY 8
of the Internet program

THE BOTTOM LINE

- ▸ So as to continue smoking, smokers lie to themselves systematically about the risks of smoking.
- ▸ Staying naive, belittling data, exercising so-called control, lying, acting overwhelmed, justifying yourself— all these are typical avoidance strategies. They cost smokers on average 10 years of their life.

16

Things Do
Get Better!

SMOKERS OFTEN SAY TO ME, "THERE'S no point in me quitting now; I've been smoking for far too long." This is not true. Often, this is only an excuse to continue smoking or fear of not managing to quit. But you will manage it if you are convinced that nicotine is of no benefit to you in terms of enjoyment, stress, or mood. And when you no longer inhale the 4,800 toxic substances, you will find enormous changes in your health and fitness.

"Exactly what changes?" Some of these toxic substances, even in the tiniest amounts, have adverse effects on your metabolism. The toxins are altering and impairing thousands of biochemical reactions of your finely tuned metabolism. They raise your heartbeat, change the stickiness of the blood platelets, reduce the disposal of degenerated cells, and so on. Large-scale studies show that due to this biochemical balance, which is so sensitive to toxic substances, smoking fewer cigarettes is of little benefit. Even the smallest amounts of these toxins have negative effects.

However, when you stop inhaling these toxins, after just one year, there is already a decrease in their negative cardiovascular effects. What you notice first of all is, of course, easier breathing. Even shortly after quitting, you can breathe more easily and don't become breathless as quickly. That really feels great and is a genuine gain on your quality of life. Quitting is worthwhile at any age and does make you more fit.

Here's what happens to you body when you stop smoking:

AFTER 20 MINUTES: Circulation improves in the hands and feet.

AFTER 2 HOURS: Pulse, heartbeat, and blood pressure normalize. In the case of pregnant women: The heartbeat of the unborn child also returns to normal.

AFTER 8 HOURS: Carbon monoxide is reduced and no longer stops oxygen from reaching the blood cells. Your cells have a much better supply of oxygen. In the case of pregnant women: Your unborn child also receives more oxygen.

AFTER 24 HOURS: Your risk of heart attack drops.

AFTER 48 HOURS: Nicotine is completely eliminated from your body.

AFTER 2 DAYS: Your sense of smell and taste improve and return.

AFTER 3 DAYS: Breathing significantly improves. The little hairs on the lungs (cilia) recover. They transport particles from the lungs. A good sign: You cough more because more and more dirt and toxic substances are being removed from the lungs.

AFTER 1 WEEK: Your blood pressure falls.

AFTER 3 MONTHS: On average lung capacity rises by 39% and shortness of breath is reduced. The skin tone also improves.

AFTER 3 TO 9 MONTHS: Smokers' cough and susceptibility to infections are reduced because the lungs can now clean themselves.

AFTER 12 MONTHS: The risk of cardiovascular disease is halved.

AFTER 5 YEARS: The risk of stomach, mouth, throat, esophageal, and lung cancer is halved.

AFTER 5 TO 10 YEARS: Depending on how much you have smoked, within this period the risk of cardiovascular diseases, heart attack, and stroke reaches the same level as that of nonsmokers.

AFTER 10 YEARS: Cell and tissue changes that were precancerous have largely been replaced. The risk of lung cancer continues to drop. The risk of cancer of the mouth, throat, esophagus, bladder, and kidneys continues to drop.

AFTER 15 YEARS: Your risk of cancer is the same as that of a nonsmoker.

THE BOTTOM LINE

▸ Not quitting because you assume it is no longer worthwhile is simply an invented excuse of an addicted brain so as to continue smoking or to counter the fear of not managing to quit.

▸ You will always benefit by ceasing to inhale toxins.

17

What Are You Going to Decide?

Decision-Making Time

Nobody needed cigarettes before slowly becoming addicted to smoking. And nobody needs cigarettes after getting rid of the addiction. In fact, nobody really decided of his or her own free will to have to smoke for the rest of his or her life. We stumble into the nicotine trap and the changes to the neurotransmitter system of the brain makes us continue smoking. At that stage, a cigarette only gets rid of an unpleasant feeling inside and brings us up to the normal level of nonsmokers. What a stupid drug, where you have to actually pay money just to feel normal, to get to a level that you had for free before you started smoking. And then after a short period of relief, you find yourself in the same trap—an endlessly repetitive chain, a vicious cycle. Do you want to continue this cycle for the rest of your life? Over time, nicotine makes you feel more nervous, susceptible to stress, and more prone to mood swings. For this "privilege," you inhale toxins that make you age prematurely, ruin your health, and shorten your life and you even pay for this. You have known for a long time how absurd this is. It gnaws away at your self-esteem that you are killing yourself because you feel you can't do without nicotine.

At the same time, the drug has conditioned many everyday situations as strong cues to make you smoke. Just like the light signal in nicotine-addicted mice causes an obsessive search for nicotine, it is as if you are remote controlled, looking for a nicotine fix in an increasing number of conditioned situations. Do you really believe that you are going to wake up one day and not want a cigarette? That is not going to happen. Because you will always want more and not less of a drug. When is the best time to quit? *Now*!

The "Now-Is-Not-the-Right-Time Trap"

Don't fall for this one: the trap that it will be easier to stop tomorrow or after one year. The trap that this is not the right time and that you should wait. This is nicotine's worst trick. It will never get easier than *now*, at *this* moment. And you've waited long enough. How many years? 10? Or maybe 20?

Let us assume that you had a glass sliver in your foot. Would you wait a few days or would you take out that sliver immediately? Or would you take out a piece of the sliver now and again to feel relief, and then step on the shard again so you could experience the additional enjoyment of pulling it out again? Your nicotine curve is exactly like this glass sliver, but in your mind. You enjoy relieving the restlessness, nervousness, and bad mood caused by the nicotine sliver. But by reaching for a cigarette, you only take the chain reaction back down to the next low nicotine level that makes you feel lousy. You force the same sliver into your mind again and again. The only option is remove the nicotine once and for all, and get rid of it. Take the sliver out of your life. Addiction has no benefits. Nicotine addiction only has disadvantages for your mind, your health, and your self-esteem. Make the decision now and fix a date to quit.

Do you want to quit?　　　　Yes ❏　　　No ❏

Money as Motivation—The Smoke Calculator

"Another price and tax rise. They're really taking us to the cleaners. If they go up again, I'm going to quit." In spite of this, you continue to smoke? How many cost increases have you seen? You are burning a fortune. Whoever smokes a pack a day is soon spending $160 to $330 a month, depending on where you live in the United States, New York City being the most expensive. That quickly adds up to $1,920 to $3,900 a year. That is equal to the price of a new computer, after just a few months, or a fantastic holiday, after one year. In the space of 40 years, you could have bought a home for the money you let go up in smoke. What would you like to buy with this money? List your genuine wishes.

1. _____

2. _____

3. _____

4. _____

5. _____

6. _____

DAY 3 OF THE INTERNET PROGRAM

THE SMOKE CALCULATOR: On this Internet page, there is a money counter that calculates how much you've spent on smoking. And when you quit, it calculates how much you'll save every week and every month. Reward yourself with this in the first weeks and months after quitting.

 THE FREE APP

"MY QUIT SMOKING COACH" You can also download our free, interactive app for IOS and Android. Of course it has a smoke calculator. But this app offers more than other apps: There is a success tracker for each smoke free day, interactive questionnaires, where you can put in your personal objectives and wishes. This app is by now the leading European-nonsmoking app. We wanted to make sure that you have a good tool with you when you are on the road and may come into a smoking situation.

Everything I Hate About Smoking

Make a list here of what disturbs you about smoking and why you want to quit.

1. _____

2. _____

3. _____

4. _____

5. _____

6. _____

7. _____

8. _____

9. _____

10. _____

 DAY 1
You can fill out this list on the website, print it out, or send it to your mobile phone so you always have it on you.

How Many of These Did You Miss Listing?

So you could only think of 5 things that you hate about smoking? That is really not enough. Here is a list of all the things that smokers have told me:

- ❏ "Feeling stressed and having a cigarette to fight it."
- ❏ "I can't get into gear in the morning without a cigarette."
- ❏ "The stench of my clothes, the upholstery, the bed-clothes, the car. It stinks everywhere."
- ❏ "My bad breath. I can't do anything about it."
- ❏ "My hair and skin smell funny. My boyfriend says everything smells of smoke."
- ❏ "Frequent periods of restlessness and dissatisfaction until I have smoked another cigarette."

❏ "Having to cough though I really wanted to laugh."

❏ "Frequent coughing while I speak or constantly coughing up phlegm . . . and my hoarse voice."

❏ "Not being able to breathe deeply and the stitch in my lungs when I take a deep breath."

❏ "Getting out of breath too quickly on the stairs or a bicycle."

❏ "Not being able to keep up with the children when we are playing and fooling around."

❏ "Feeling exhausted even after the slightest physical exertion."

❏ "A burning feeling in my stomach because of too much acid."

❏ "I often lose the sense of feeling in my fingertips. It makes me panic."

❏ "Constant colds in winter, which turn into bronchitis."

❏ "Headaches in the morning and smoking to get rid of them."

❏ "The constant taste of ash and toxins in my mouth."

❏ "My yellowish skin, fingers, and fingernails. Circles under my eyes. I feel ugly. Dry and wrinkled skin."

❏ "The constant fear of what I am doing to my health. I don't even go to the doctor anymore."

❏ "I constantly fight against these images of lung cancer. That takes up so much of my energy. I feel awful when I smoke but can't stop."

❏ "Fear not to be able to perform sexually."

❏ "A constant feeling of dissatisfaction and a bad mood when I can't smoke."

❏ "To become stressed later because I've wasted time to stand smoking outside the door."

❏ "My nonsmoking colleagues' thinking that I work less because I smoke."

❏ "What people are saying behind my back when I am smoking outside the door again."

- ❏ "Having to drive to the gas station late at night. I hate this feeling of compulsion."
- ❏ "To be on the edge of a nervous breakdown when the cigarette machine gets jammed."
- ❏ "Having to bum a cigarette from others."
- ❏ "At night, when I pull a half-smoked butt from the ashtray, to light again. That's really humiliating."
- ❏ "When my cigarette falls on the floor when I am driving, or even worse, when it burns a hole in the seat of the car."
- ❏ "Ash all over my trousers or on a friend's carpet."
- ❏ "Ashtrays full to the brim, which I have to carry away."
- ❏ "Having to get a nicotine fix on the balcony when it's raining."
- ❏ "Interrupting a flirtation because I am becoming increasingly nervous and can't think of anything else besides a few puffs of a cigarette."
- ❏ "Feeling too weak to stop. It is ridiculous because I know that I am killing myself."
- ❏ "I hate feeling like I have to smoke when I have a cup of coffee and I have to scrounge one up."
- ❏ "This is absurd, but because of my dog I smoke on the balcony. If he became ill, I could never forgive myself."
- ❏ "What my children think of me. Whether they will start smoking."
- ❏ "I have such a bad conscience. What happens if I become ill? Who will take care of the children?"
- ❏ "I travel a lot. I hate trembling fingers during a long train journey or after a 10-hour flight. Then, like a drug addict, going to a smoking room or the smoker's zone on the railway platform."
- ❏ "That smoking does not show strength of character. At work I try never to smoke when I have clients. That's not always easy."

❏ "Yellow wallpaper, those signs of toxins, and the smell of old smoke at home."

❏ "Getting smoke from my own cigarettes in my eyes."

❏ "Getting on other people's nerves when the wind is blowing in the wrong direction. It always seems to blow in the wrong direction."

❏ "Nonsmokers getting on my nerves with their stupid comments."

❏ "Those looks when I feed my addiction outside the door."

❏ "Losing concentration when I can´t have a cigarette."

❏ "The feeling of everything getting on my nerves faster until I can have another cigarette."

❏ "Not to singe anyone in the clubs, if you can still smoke there."

❏ "Getting ash in my drink. So what? I drink it anyway."

❏ "The constant fear of not quitting early enough and having to undergo painful therapy."

❏ "Constantly washing clothes smelling of smoke, as well as smelling it in my long hair."

❏ "Burning money every day and ruining my health at the same time."

❏ "Having a bad taste in my mouth before a good meal."

❏ "Long meetings or family celebrations where I can't smoke."

❏ "Having to put on lipstick again after each cigarette."

❏ "Having to lower the window in the car when it is raining, so I can smoke."

❏ "Trying to get rid of cigarette ash out of the car window when driving."

❏ "To stink like an ashtray in the morning and the disgusted look from my boyfriend."

❏ "Quickly arranging for some chewing gum before kissing."

❏ "Not feeling attractive to others. For nonsmokers to show no interest in me."

❏ "After sex, leaving a warm bed to disappear onto the balcony."

❏ "My friends have expensive holidays in really expensive resorts and I waste my money on cigarettes."

❏ "I buy cheap food so I have money for cigarettes"

❏ "My children would really love to go to a park or have us do something together. Instead of that, I buy cigarettes for myself and then say we haven't got enough money. I feel really awful."

Your new life as a nonsmoker is so much simpler when cigarettes don't rule your life. You'll never miss all these unpleasant situations or long for them. After a short time, you'll feel more balanced, calmer, and less stressed. You will soon feel freer and fitter. Quite apart from your feeling of pride that you've once and for all escaped the lethal toxic trap.

Setting the Date for Freedom

Choose a fixed date in the calendar. It should be at least 2 but not more than 10 days away.

❏ If you set a date more than 10 days ahead, your motivation decreases, and before you know it, you find an excuse that *now* is not the right time.

❏ If it is less than 2 days, you don't have enough time to prepare and to finish reading this book in peace. There are important chapters that could help you concerning nicotine patches, hypnosis, and antismoking medications. Don't miss the chapter about weight and whether smokers are really slimmer than nonsmokers. Read how sweets can maintain nicotine addiction, in addition to getting lots of practical advice on how to hold your weight down without dieting. Take your time to read these chapters.

❏ For premenopausal women: Set the quitting date in the first 15 days following your period, particularly if you have greater mood swings during your period. It has been shown that women have fewer withdrawal symptoms and depressive moods are less common if you stop during the first 15 days after your period than if you stop 15 days directly before having your period.[93] Here, quitting smoking overlaps more with the effects of the period, when bad moods are more common.

❏ Decide to stop on a day when you don't have a lot of stress, but at the same time you will have some distractions. This varies for everyone.

❏ If you're always stressed at work, then stop during a weekend. Decide to do something on the day you quit, preferably with your best nonsmoker friend. Do something you enjoy and that distracts you.

❏ If you have more stress at home with your family than at work, then stop on a working day. But remember you may be a little edgy on this day and could have difficulty concentrating.

Write your quitting day into your calendar. Look forward to it. Tell your friends, so you don't change your mind.

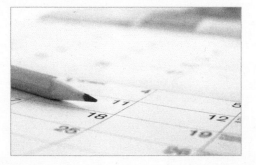

The Cigarette Butt Museum

Open a cigarette-butt museum from now until you stop smoking: Empty your ashtray into 2 lidded jars. Keep a large glass jar for home and a smaller one for when you are out, a little one that will fit into every handbag or pocket. Your sense of smell will improve by the end of the first day you stop smoking. When you feel like a cigarette, first have a smell of the cigarette-butt museum. That will put an end to the idea right away. Believe me, this is incredibly effective!

The Most Important Rule: Never Question Your Decision!

Of course you're afraid that you won't manage to quit. But you've uncovered the nicotine trap and will succeed like millions of other smokers. Finish this book in the coming days. You've just decided to liberate yourself from the toxic smoke prison!

 CONGRATULATIONS! You have just earned your third star for mastering the tough parts of the book on topics that you avoided in the past. And, you've made a decision. You have come a very long way!

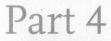

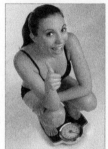

Part 4

Become a Nonsmoker and Maintain Your Weight

18

Smoking Doesn't Keep You Slim

SMOKING MAKES YOU UNATTRACTIVE. And being at your desired weight is only a small part of what makes you attractive! All the same, no one wants to put on an excessive amount of weight after quitting smoking. Although other withdrawal symptoms such as lack of concentration, irritability, and moodiness already improve after 2 weeks from your quitting date, the withdrawal symptom "phantom hunger" lingers for another 3 to 4 months. Unless you want to gain weight, you will have to take a conscious and deliberate approach to the problem of withdrawal hunger. Online and in almost all books on quitting smoking, the problem of phantom hunger and weight gain is played down or you find trivial tips, such as, "Eat more fruit and vegetables." But playing this down is no solution when smokers fail to quit on account of it. So, let's face the problem!

"Keep On Smoking, It Keeps You Slim."

192

For over a fifth of all male smokers and one third of all female smokers, the fear of putting on weight is a reason for leaving things the way they are and not trying to quit. After not smoking for several weeks, many grab a cigarette out of fear of putting on more weight.[94, 95]

An addicted brain jumps at every opportunity. Mercilessly! And it will whisper to you, "Keep on smoking, it keeps you slim;" "Do you really want to keep on gaining weight?" "Just one little cigarette can't hurt—you're going to feel hungry for the rest of your life, if you don't," or "Just going to enjoy a little treat, a smoke, and the hunger will be gone and everything will be okay weight-wise." Does any of this ring a bell? Don't be deceived. Cigarettes don´t keep you slim. And smokers who've put on weight while trying to quit aren't going to lose it again simply by reverting to their old smoking habits. This is another lame excuse to start smoking again.

Cigarettes don´t do anything for you in terms of weight management. On the contrary: Smoking and the resulting distorted metabolism in your body are the real reason that you put on weight when you quit.

A Myth—Smoking Does Not Keep You Slim

For over 30 years, cigarette advertising has been promoting that cigarettes keep you slim. After the US government prohibited these advertising lies in the 1950s, such brands as Virginia Slims came on the market, using particularly slim models. The cigarette industry bought its way into Hollywood productions big time on account of advertising restrictions. Slim smoking stars in films and television series are unbeatable role models. A slender, smoking fashion icon, such as Sarah Jessica Parker in *Sex in the City*, is

Nonsmokers Don't Have More Excess Weight Than Smokers

worth her weight in gold. Equally dumb are the remarks made by prattling pop stars about cigarettes and staying slim. But it works: The fact is, 66.4% of girls in grades 9 through 12 smoke specifically so as to lose weight.[96]

Nonsmokers Do Not Weigh More Than Smokers

So, does smoking really make or keep you slim? Let's expose the lie. Just a few examples: A study conducted on the body weight of 55,000 women over a period of 8 years shows that female nonsmokers didn't put on more weight than female smokers did.[97] Interesting! And in the case of 5,115 smokers of both genders between the ages of 18 and 30, over a period of 7 years, no weight differences could be determined between smokers and nonsmokers.[98] But the myth of slim smokers gets even shakier: A girl going through puberty doesn't smoke with the idea of looking slimmer than her current girlfriends in 30 years' time. Still young people succumb to the false promises made by slim, smoking film and pop idols. We hold on to this superstition as an unshakeable truth to justify smoking throughout our smoking career.

But smoking doesn't keep you slim. In fact, there are even studies that show that smokers put on *more* weight than nonsmokers do. A 5-year study of 7,500 Spanish students demonstrates this. [99] Study after study has proven that smoking causes unattractive fat redistribution. The latest study measured the dimensions of 21,000 male and female smokers bodies.[100] Smoking caused changes in their sugar and fat metabolism and made them more likely to put on weight than nonsmokers.

Smoking Causes Metabolic Changes and Makes You Fat

An increase in abdominal fat is only a symptom that something has changed for the worse in the metabolism. Smoking causes insulin resistance. This means that insulin—the hormone responsible for storing sugar—no longer works the way it should, and can cause diabetes over time. Smoking doubles the risk of becoming diabetic.

But what does insulin resistance have to do with putting on weight after you quit smoking? Insulin stores sugar in fat cells, but as long as there is plenty of insulin in the bloodstream, this energy won't be released. What is conceived as a "temporary energy storage facility" becomes a "permanent spare tire storage site." If you become resistant to insulin, your body must constantly produce additional insulin, as it isn't functioning as well as it should. This also means that you will constantly have an excess of insulin circulating in your bloodstream and that the sugar is going only in one direction—to be stored in the fat cells of the oddly expanding abdominal area of smokers.

But because smokers burn some additional 200 calories daily through other changes in their metabolism, they don't put on weight as long as they smoke, even though the unsightly redistribution of body fat is already apparent. This has been demonstrated by a study of 21,000 smokers.

Insulin resistance really shows its full effects when you quit smoking. Ex-smokers, through their constantly high insulin levels, have little access to the fat deposits as sources of energy and instead store more sugar in their fat cells.

"Well, I didn't really want to know about that in such glorious detail." That's clear. But it's important to know that the so-called "I stay slim cigarettes" are the *cause* of these changes in the metabolism, which then cause you to put on weight when you first quit smoking. Now the good news: This insulin resistance and other metabolic changes recede again in ex-smokers.[101] But this can easily take a year. And that's if you don't already have diabetes, as insulin resistance is also the preliminary stage of diabetes. The earlier you quit, the greater your chances are of ridding yourself of insulin resistance. Working out also helps to regenerate the metabolism more quickly, as it makes the cells sensitive to insulin again. After about one year, ex-smokers rarely continue to gain weight. After 2 years, many ex-smokers regained their former weight and their metabolism had returned to normal. So a long-term strategic plan is needed here. Quitting smoking is a game of strategy.

You're Fat Because You Smoke

It's clearly a myth that smoking makes or keeps you slim. Cigarettes are the real reason why you put on weight when you quit smoking. Your metabolism had been altered by nicotine. If you hadn't started smoking in the first place, you wouldn't be faced with this problem. It's the same story with stress. Smoking doesn't reduce stress—it causes it. Be careful not to confuse cause and effect. Take a long, cold look at the situation: You don't put on weight because you quit smoking. You put on weight because you smoked in the past. Smoking is of no advantage if you want to stay slim; smokers are statistically no slimmer, even if cigarette-sponsored Hollywood tries to make us believe the opposite. On the contrary, cigarettes are the very reason why you put on weight when you quit due to your changed metabolism. With a few nutritional tricks and exercising a bit more, you will find a way out of this metabolic smoking trap and you won't put on weight.

The Myth of Gaining 20 Pounds When You Quit Smoking

It's a fallacy! 43 studies showed that weight increase on average is 6.17 pounds.[102] Anyone can deal with that. What's interesting to note is that overall weight increase ranged from 1.76 to 17.6 pounds. The smokers who gained the most weight were those that had always had weight fluctuations and exercised the least.

Is that a surprise? Even a little common sense tells us that people who eat healthy only now and again and are couch potatoes will also experience a yo-yo effect when they quit smoking. So, dear slim smokers: Don't worry so much about quitting smoking! Your weight will not mushroom.

You Don't Need to Worry About Your Diet or Exercise—The Fears of Overweight Smokers

Smokers who are a little overweight and have quite a bit of experience with dieting have a great fear of putting on weight.[103] In a large survey, 40% of female smokers who had frequently gone on diets and generally had a higher body weight stated that they started to smoke again when they realized they had gained weight after quitting.[104] If this is the way you think, then there is one thing you should always keep in mind: The weight increase is a temporary phenomenon. And it doesn't mean you have to put on a lot of weight. Please read this chapter twice and convince yourself that continuing to smoke will in no way keep you slimmer in the long term.

With or without cigarettes, with the wrong diet you'll always continue to put on weight. So take the first step toward a healthier life. Use this new energy in your life to become more physically active. Soon you will feel fitter without cigarettes. Maybe you will exercise more. This will keep your weight in much better check than continuing to smoke and feeling out of breath so quickly, not getting enough oxygen for more energy, feeling too tired to do anything, and lying around on the couch. Get out of the house. Spend the money you save from not smoking on a bicycle or on visiting a fitness center. Cigarettes won't make you slim, although you have convinced yourself otherwise. They'll only make you lazy and sick.

You'll Get Back to Your Normal Weight

Once again: Studies show that most ex-smokers return to their normal weight after 2 years. And if you do put on some weight in the beginning, you will lose it again later, after you've become a stable nonsmoker. Think of all the advantages for the way you look. In spite of all your concerns about putting on weight, don't make the classic mistake: Do not quit smoking and experiment at the same time with keeping your weight down by eating less. This just causes too much stress all together and will doom your attempts to failure. You need to feel satisfied and full to score your first victory over nicotine. Look at the slight increase in weight as something temporary until your metabolism has regenerated itself.

Why Does Smoking Make You Feel Less Hungry?

Nicotine docks directly onto the appetite control center of the brain. Through additional docking areas (receptors) in the brain, it leads to the release of a neurotransmitter called dopamine. You met this before. Dopamine also controls the appetite. The more dopamine there is in the brain, the less hungry you feel.

"But that must make smokers slimmer." It doesn't. When the nicotine level in the blood falls after 30 minutes and your neurotransmitter for happiness is also reduced, then the feeling of hunger returns with a vengeance. So you start to eat even more. As a result, the actual effect is that smokers are *not* slimmer than nonsmokers.

Lighting Up to Avoid Feeling Hungry

That empty, hungry feeling is similar to your desire for a cigarette. By eating or smoking a cigarette, you want to feel better. Both eating and smoking influence the neurotransmitters in the brain that make you feel satisfied. Many people unconsciously smoke to suppress their feeling of being hungry. At work, when you are too busy to eat, is a good example. Many cigarettes are smoked just to put off that hungry feeling. This is an illusion, as later in the day, the body will get the calories it needs. So, when you quit smoking, be prepared again for the totally natural hunger signals from your body when your cells require an energy boost. Many smokers are no longer aware of these natural hunger cycles because they have manipulated them for 20 to 30 years by using cigarettes to stop feeling hungry and to repress this feeling. Look forward to the return of this healthy and natural bodily need.

The Natural Hunger Cycle

Your addicted brain will lead you to believe for some time that you are hungry once you have quit smoking. Only too well do I know this empty feeling in my stomach. But this, too, will pass in a few weeks, as soon as the neurotransmitter processes in the brain have returned to normal.

But how can you tell normal hunger from withdrawal hunger? Let me tell you about my good friend Brigitte. She smoked a pack a day for 10 years, particularly in the late afternoon and in the evening—when she was at home and felt alone—probably because the fridge was usually empty and she was trying to rid herself of hunger systematically through smoking. One Saturday, we were out and about in the city. She had quit smoking 3 weeks previously. "Without a cigarette I have this constant feeling of hunger, now, once again," Brigitte said. She hadn't noticed that she had last eaten something 6 hours earlier and that her hunger was perfectly normal at that time. In the past, quite unconsciously, she had lit one cigarette after the other to "smoke away" her hunger. She no longer knew the natural feeling of nonsmokers that energy requires regular refueling. First, I had to retrain her think-ing that she really wasn't suffering a withdrawal symptom but that her body cells were simply crying, "We need more energy, please refuel." The feeling of hunger cannot always be equated with needing a cigarette. Adding up the snacks in between, it is quite normal to eat 4 to 5 times a day. Give yourself a little time to get used to this natural hunger cycle. Perhaps you've been manipulating this for decades, since you were 13 or 14.

Why Do You Put On Weight When You Quit Smoking and What Can You Do About It?

Nicotine accelerates various metabolic processes and leads, for example, to the secretion of the stress hormone adrenaline. This increases the rate at which fat is burned. If you're smoking to burn the fat off, you are really just keeping yourself in an unnecessary state of constant stress.

Smoking is also the cause of other metabolic changes. As a result, smokers burn some 200 calories more daily than do non-smokers.[105] "Great. For sure, that must keep my weight down," your addicted brain answers immediately. Once again: Statistically, smokers are not slimmer than nonsmokers (see page 193). The temporary weight gain when you quit is caused by "overeating" when your very real hunger that has been artifi-cially repressed by nicotine eventually breaks through and craves satisfaction.

But you can easily shed those additional 200 calories by using just a few tricks: a little more physical exercise, no-calorie sweet-eners instead of sugar, more fruit to fight the little pangs of hun-ger, a little less fat consumption, and more protein to feel full. That alone will do the trick. It is easy and *it is not a diet.*

THE BOTTOM LINE: CIGARETTES NEITHER MAKE YOU SLIM NOR MORE ATTRACTIVE.

Ouch . . . so much work to persuade the addicted brain. I hope I convinced you 100%:

- ► Cigarettes don't keep you slim, but make you less attractive.
- ► Smokers do not weigh less than nonsmokers.
- ► By smoking, you manipulate your feeling of hunger but do not eat less.
- ► Cigarettes cause metabolic changes that do make you gain weight just after you first quit.
- ► You don't put on weight because you quit smoking. You put on weight because you have been a smoker!

19

Addiction and the Sweet Tooth

Why Does Nicotine Withdrawal Make You Want to Eat Something Sweet?

For a long time, it was not understood why smokers who quit develop an irresistible urge to eat sweet things, thus putting on weight. Only in 2004 was it demonstrated that sugar in the body leads to the rapid release of dopamine and other neurotransmitters.[106][107][108]

So, it is more than logical: When the nicotine-based dopamine kick is missing, smokers will try to replace this reward mechanism with a sweetness-based dopamine kick. And before you fall back into your old way of thinking—"You see? Smoking really does reward me with dopamine"—once again: what is really happening is that nicotine causes the receptors in the brain to become less sensitive. That is the only reason you need more nicotine or sweets: to stimulate the neurotransmitter for more happiness, so that you can attain even just the normal reward and satisfaction level of a nonsmoker! There is no dopamine-edge advantage to smoking; it is the cause of your problem. The neurotransmitters want their accustomed fix, and if nicotine isn't coming, maybe sweets will do the trick.

The desire for sweets proves the following: Those who have given up smoking do not put on weight because they no longer smoke or because smoking kept them slim; they put on weight because they smoked previously. When the neurotransmitter system becomes normalized to no longer depend on nicotine to release dopamine, binge eating will go away and there will be no further increase in weight. You just have to go through this once.

Obesity—The Big Sugar Dopamine Binge

In many how-to-quit books, you can read: "Eat as little sugar as possible." Apart from calories and weight increase, what is behind that? One of the most exciting new discoveries is that many obese individuals compulsively shovel sugar into themselves just to get a dopamine kick. They manipulate their mood and feeling of well-being with sugar and condition themselves, just like smokers, in an increasing number of situations to give themselves a dopamine kick to improve their mood. Whoever compulsively and constantly devours sugar develops amazing changes in the brain, and in the neurotransmitter system in particular, which lead to withdrawal symptoms if sugar is not forthcoming. If there is no sugar replenishment, this leads to feelings of nervousness, dissatisfaction, and even fear, because the brain has become used to such a strong release of dopamine.[109] [110]

Sugar—More Addictive Than Cocaine

Sugar can lead to a stronger dependency than cocaine. You think I am exaggerating? Prof. Serge Ahmed, of the University of

Bordeaux, is one of the leading specialists in the area of the brain and addiction. He discovered that when rats have the choice between sugar and cocaine, 90% of them choose sugar rather than cocaine to get the body's dopamine kick.[111]

And this has astonished scientists as well: Even rats addicted to cocaine prefer sugar. Not even light electroshocks can stop them from sucking on sugar, so strong is the urge for it. Something else interesting to note about such experiments: in sugar withdrawal one can detect exactly the same neurotransmitters for stress and fear as in the case of drug withdrawal.[112] Even after 2 weeks of withdrawal, the little rodents return to excessive overconsumption of sugar. Research into the sugar-dopamine addiction cycle shows that this can even reach addiction levels, as we know from the case of sugar-dependent obese individuals. These are people who literally eat themselves to death through the compulsive eating of sweets. But then, who among us has not sometimes taken solace in chocolate or candy. Science is only describing something we already do. Each of us has run to the corner shop to get that little sugar-dopamine kick. We walk for miles not just for Camel but also for Mars and Snickers and . . .

Becoming Fat and Relapsing Due to Sugar

What is the point of looking at the relationship between sugar and addiction in such detail, in a book about smoking? Because you need to be careful not to simply replace nicotine with sugar when you quit. Smokers clearly have the urge to compensate with something other than nicotine to get their accustomed dopamine reward and manipulate their mood. But this leaves them precisely in the same addiction cycle: First, they put on a large amount of weight when they fill up on sugar to get their dopamine kick. Second, the receptors in the brain and the neurotransmitters recover at a slower rate. One can see from animal experiments with sugar that the changes in the receptors in the brain are similar to those of drug addicts. [113] [114] [115] It is no coincidence that many ex-smokers who have gotten used to the dopamine-replacement sugar overconsumption, and who have put on a lot of weight as a result, are more likely to relapse.

Many stories run like this: "After putting on 20 pounds, I preferred to go back to smoking." However, it is not really the weight that causes people to start smoking again; rather, their feelings of dissatisfaction because the insensitive receptors in the brain have not recovered sufficiently and needed to get lots dopamine to get them in a normal state of well-being. It's important to see through this! Do not fall victim to this displaced addiction cycle. It will not get you off cigarettes but traps you right back there with a renewed desire for nicotine or sweet substitute satisfaction.

MY ADVICE: Eating something sweet now and again when the nicotine craving hits you to get a dopamine fix is okay. You can also use a no-calorie sweetener for this (see pages 217–18), which works just as well. The rodents in the experiment got the same dopamine fix [116] with artificial sugar as with sugar, but at least without calories. Why does that happen? The signal for "sweet," not for sugar specifically, is what causes the brain to release the neurotransmitters. Whoever falls into this trap of the sugar-dopamine-consumption-cycle by consuming sugary or fatty sweets can easily gain an extra 20 pounds instead of the average of 6 that ex-smokers put on when quitting smoking—and the addiction behavior still remains. So, moderate your sugar intake, replace the sugar with no-calorie sweeteners, and keep tabs on your weight gain. From sugar-packed yogurts to coffee with sugar—you really can find palatable substitutes for this unnecessary substance. More details on sugar are to be found on pages 208–210. Try as much as possible not to satisfy your cravings for nicotine with sugar. You'll only be comforting yourself with a displaced addiction cycle.

THE BOTTOM LINE

- ► Nicotine causes changes in the receptors in the brain that make you feel less rewarded and satisfied.
- ► Smokers who quit replace nicotine with sugar to enhance their mood by means of a dopamine fix.
- ► Sugar causes the same changes as drugs in the transmitter substances of the brain.
- ► By consuming too many sweets, not only do you put on weight but you run greater chances of relapsing.
- ► Sugar substitutes provide a dopamine fix without the calories.

20

How to Avoid the Roly-Poly Trap

Happiness and Eating

Here, we've arrived at the beautiful side of life—eating. A few days after you quit smoking, your sense of taste starts to improve. Of course, that makes you feel like eating more. Next to sex, eating is a great life-affirming act compared to smoking. For many, eating is the sex of old age. Well, I'm not completely convinced of that—but food provides not only bodily pleasure—it is a cultural and social activity. Enjoy it!

With good food, you are refueling your 70 billion body cells with vitality. Get your metabolism in shape again. Metabolism is nothing more than the body's changing food into energy, hormones, and happiness, to give but 3 examples. And that is exactly what I want you to experience: more vitality, more energy, a better feeling of well-being. And all this without putting on weight.

"But how much could I eat without gaining weight?" A lot! You will be amazed at just how much! The most important thing in keeping your weight stable is to feel full and satisfied. Whoever feels hungry cannot keep his or her weight. Whoever is hungry will try to find consolation in chocolate and other things that cause a yo-yo effect on poundage.

Dieting Is Depressing—Food Makes You Happy

A diet represents discipline, hunger, frustration, giving something up, a bad conscience, and defeat. And that is the last thing you need—you have enough to deal with just getting off nicotine. You need to fill up with biomolecules that stimulate vitality and well-being. "And just how is that supposed to happen?" For this you need magnesium, B vitamins, and protein. Both magnesium and the B vitamins are particularly active in the nervous system. Magnesium calms and relaxes the whole nervous system. A slight lack of both of these substances can make you feel nervous and on edge. So, it is a good idea to supplement these for a few weeks.

But, of course, we were talking about enjoyment. It's more fun eating to get these benefits. You can get all the nutrients you need from tasty fruits, vegetables, protein from lean meat, and, above all, low–calorie, high-protein shakes.

The 4 Building Blocks to Keep Your Figure and Be Happy

Here are the 4 building blocks you need to maintain your weight and stay energetic in the coming weeks.

EAT FEWER QUICK CARBOHYDRATES TO AVOID THE INSULIN-HUNGER TRAP. Rapidly digested and absorbed carbohydrates, just like cigarettes, give you a short-lived fix. Then you quickly feel hungry again, due to low glucose levels, and you'll want more quick carbohydrates. This up and down of your energy level makes you unhappy and fat.

11. **EAT MORE FRUITS AND VEGETABLES—GREATER VOLUME, FEWER CALORIES.** These really make you feel full, and with each passing day, the vitamins and minerals will make you feel more energetic. Instead of inhaling 4,000 toxic substances, you are beginning a new life. Important: You always feel as well as your metabolism functions. So refuel regularly with these vital substances.

12. **EAT MORE PROTEIN, TO FEEL FULLER AND HAPPIER.** This is how you avoid the hunger attacks caused by nicotine withdrawal. Protein sends a feeling of fullness to the brain. Frustration is driven off as protein increases the brain's happiness neurotransmitter production—protein is the raw material to build these neurotransmitters.

13. **KEEP PHYSICALLY ACTIVE, TO FIGHT OFF LITTLE ADDICTION ATTACKS.** Exercise keeps your weight down. There is nothing new about that. Over the long term, exercise will counter withdrawal attacks and cravings because it, too, leads to a release of happiness neurotransmitters.

Similarities of the Sugar and the Nicotine Trap

One thing you already know: Smokers reach for Candy & Co as a replacement for smoking. If you start with chocolate bars, you will easily walk straight into the sugar trap, which works very similarly to the nicotine trap. Once you start on sweets, you will need to top off again every 30 to 45 minutes; otherwise you'll become grumpy, nervous, and feel hungry again. In this way, you'll eat yourself into a hunger cycle: becoming increasingly hungry, you will become increasingly dependent on getting your next sugar fix and you will put on more and more weight.

How does this work? When you eat foods rich in sugar or other rapidly absorbed carbohydrates, such as potatoes or white bread, the energy is released much too quickly into the bloodstream. This energy cannot be completely used up, and a chain reaction begins: Once in the system, the energy needs someplace to go temporarily. Insulin, the sugar-storage hormone, places the superfluous energy in the fat cells—for emergencies. When your energy detectors signal that a massive amount of sugar has just been delivered, then the body releases a large amount of insulin. Due to the high levels of insulin now circulating in the body, too much sugar is placed into storage, and after a short time you have too little sugar in your blood. Your blood sugar level now becomes too low—you're hypoglycemic. At the same time, energy-providing fat cannot be released from the fat cells as long as there is insulin in your blood. So the energy is trapped in the fat cells. That is why your metabolism, particularly your brain, which functions on sugar, is screaming, "I need more sugar, pronto! I'm quite nervous and grumpy because of a lack of sugar!" The next bar of chocolate or soft drink does the trick ensuring that your energy is bumped up . . . but overdoes it.

And so, you swing to and fro every 40-odd minutes: *too low blood sugar level . . . eat something sweet . . . short-term satisfaction and sugar fix . . . sugar is stored away . . . a hunger and nervousness due to low blood sugar . . . impulsive bumping up with more sugar.* This process makes you eat more and feel hungrier.

This may remind you of the nicotine cycle: *lack of nicotine . . . smoking to counteract this . . . getting the short-term nicotine fix . . . a quick breakdown of nicotine . . . leading to a nervous restlessness and a feeling of emptiness . . . bumping up with more nicotine.*

The similarities over time and the symptoms are striking: nervous, stressed, and requiring another hit. And, when you have devoured a bar of chocolate or gotten your nicotine fix, the predominant temporary feeling is of relief. But that relief is woefully short-lived, and then the whole cycle begins again.

Overweight on Account of Hunger

Once it gets started, you can go through this sugar-driven hunger cycle a dozen times a day. It is the main reason for being overweight. I remember a female cashier who was very overweight, sitting with a bottle of Coca-Cola at the register. She topped up with Coca-Cola again and again throughout the day. A 36-ounce bottle of Coca-Cola contains 28 cubes of sugar or a whopping 9 tablespoons. When I asked her about it she said, "Yes, but I'm hungry." And, that is exactly the point I want to make. If you feel constant hunger, you cannot keep your original weight. If there is one basic rule, then it is the following: *Whoever wants to stay slim must feel they have eaten well.*

Whoever wants to remain slim must feel full. The sugar trap is just like the nicotine trap. With quick carbohydrates, you just get hungrier and more nervous.

And note the emotional similarity between those who are overweight and those who are in the nicotine trap: It often starts with a negative feeling that you want to counter: *consume sugar . . . short-term satisfaction . . . hunger attack . . . frustration . . . turning again to sugar, to feel better . . . feelings of guilt.*

So, How Do You Escape from the Sugar Trap?

Do you know the secret to staying slim? It's your insulin level. It must remain as low as possible. Fruit, vegetables, and whole-grain products cause the insulin level to remain low as energy is

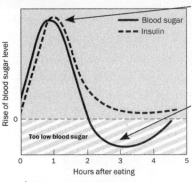

Quick energy

Hunger due to low blood sugar level

What is the secret of staying slim?
You consume slow energy: foods that are slowly digested—lots of fiber, vegetables, and protein. The result: less unneeded quick energy is stored in the fat cells.

How do you burn more fat?
"Slow" energy makes you feel full for a long time. It does not cause a low blood sugar level. The body just switches to burning fat and you get hungry hours later.

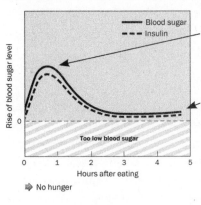

Slow energy

No hunger

How do the calories land in your belly zone?
"Fast" energy makes you fat. The energy reaches the bloodstream too quickly. The sugar storage hormone, insulin, is released and stores unneeded energy in the fat cells.

Why do you become hungry faster?
Due to the high release of insulin, too much energy is transported into your fat cells. The consequence: low blood sugar. That's why you get hungry faster and eat more. With quick carbs, you eat yourself into a cycle where you get more and more hungry and gain weight. Only when you feel full for a longer time can you maintain your weight or lose weight.

released slowly into the bloodstream. It is because of fiber in such foods that energy gets into the blood less quickly. In addition, fructose, the natural sugars in fruit, keeps the insulin level relatively stable. With protein and fats the insulin level stays completely flat. In fact, you can lose weight on a diet of proteins and fats due to its low insulin level. The Atkins diet is a good example of this.

How does that work? Whenever energy is slowly released into the bloodstream, very little insulin is released. Later, the body switches the fuel automatically and starts to burn fat again. Only when there is no insulin in the blood is the fat released from the fat cells. So, more and more fat leaves the cells and becomes part of the energy mix. When you burn fat, you don't feel hungry. As a result, you eat less. You don't get nervous or fidgety and your weight remains stable because you feel full.

This Is How You Remain Calm and Feel Full

The glycemic index indicates how quickly the energy from a particular food reaches the bloodstream. In fact, it is simple common sense. You do not need a long nutrition list to select the best choices for you. Quick energy is supplied by food that

- has gone through a lot of processing
- is rich in sugar
- contains little fiber

It is as simple as that. Potatoes (little fiber), processed grains, as in toasted bread (little fiber), sweets (sugar), soft drinks (sugar), all manufactured products (sugar and little fiber) cause this sugar-hunger curve. In contrast, milk products (provided they are not sugared), whole-grain products (a lot of fiber), and fruit (fiber and natural fruit sugar) keep the insulin curve stable. Meat and vegetables keep the insulin curve completely flat and stable.

Our old metabolic software, the product of millions of years of human evolution, is not adapted to quick energy. This kind of quick energy just never existed in the wild. Instead, fiber-rich foods and protein were consumed. It has only been over the past 100 years that people have become fatter and hungrier because the quick energy is being shoveled too fast from our ancient insulin program into our fat cells and this lack of sugar causes hunger. Former smokers who change over to consuming more natural foods no longer fall into the insulin-hunger-trap and feel full for a long time. Only those who eat until they feel full or satisfied remain slim.

The Fatal Nicotine Sugar Trap

As the feeling of hunger is so similar to that of nicotine withdrawal, you'll have frequent mini-feeding frenzies and a sweet tooth. That's no problem if you satisfy this phantom hunger with chewing gum or fruit, or eat to be full with your regular meals.

> Pangs of hunger caused by low blood sugar can heighten the desire for cigarettes.

If, however, instead of that, you fall into the hunger trap and calm the cigarette withdrawal hunger with sugary gum drops, you will end up in a further withdrawal cycle. You won't just be trying to calm the phantom hunger, which doesn't work anyway, but, in addition, you'll be eating away every 30 to 45 minutes to fight the lack of sugar in your bloodstream. With quick carbohydrates you'll become fatter and fatter and increasingly hungry and nervous. For years you've trained yourself to manipulate and suppress this nervous hungry feeling by smoking cigarettes. This impulse to smoke is programmed in your brain. But be careful! This fatal combination of hunger, low levels of sugar in the bloodstream, nervousness and dissatisfaction can all too easily increase the desire for a cigarette. And, on top of that you will start to devour more and more sweets. And, continue to put on weight. The nicotine-sugar-traps spring shut: *intake of sugar – short-lived feeling of satisfaction – hunger attack – top up with sugar – feelings of guilt on account of weight gain – hunger/frustration/feeling nervous – increasing longing for cigarettes to fill the void.*

Fruits and Vegetables—High in Volume but Low in Calories

Fruits and vegetables not only keep the insulin level stable but will give you a feeling of being full by means of one simple mechanism: you eat a high volume of them. They are bulky and take up a lot of space in the stomach. The stomach is then full, with very few calories to show for it. Stretch stimuli make you feel full. "Hey, stop! There's no more room," the stomach says. Make use of this. If you start with a salad, you'll eat less of the main course without wasting a thought over it.

Exactly the opposite is true for fat. Fat crams as many calories as possible in the smallest space. The feeling of being full is transmitted too late to the brain and by that time you've already consumed 200 to 300 calories too much. Eat as much fruit or vegetables as you want. They won't make you fat.

Do Heavy Smokers Like Milk and Fruit?

A cigarette after eating an apple. Yuck—what a terrible taste. Drink a glass of milk and smoke—even worse. Every fifth smoker says that after milk or fruit, a cigarette tastes bad.[117] Do yourself a favor: Should you ever have a relapse, drink some milk before you light up a cigarette. It will taste really disgusting. The opposite also holds true. If you've been a chain-smoker throughout your life, it may well be that you rarely ate milk products or fruit. But without cigarettes, your ability to taste will change. Those who quit smoking often begin to like the taste of milk products and fruit again. One advantage: Both food groups are not coupled to the "satisfying feeling" of a cigarette, the way coffee or alcohol are.

Give it a try.

My Advice on Fighting Hunger Attacks

CHEW AS MUCH SUGAR-FREE CHEWING GUM AS YOU CAN. Gum is sweet, keeps the insulin level stable, and keeps your mouth occupied. There are many different flavors to choose from.

EAT AS MUCH FRUIT AS POSSIBLE. Eating fruit has a lot to do with its simply being there. You have to have it in the house. In addition, never leave the house without a banana or an apple in your handbag or backpack. Do you take fruit with you to work? Do it! Have you packed fruit for the lengthy car journey? Make sure you have it with you. Under no circumstances should you stop at the next convenience store and buy a bar of chocolate because you feel hungry . . . and then end up with a pack of cigarettes in your hands. Always have fruit within reach during the first week of quitting smoking.

YOU CAN MAKE A FRUIT SALAD IN THE TIME IT TAKES TO SMOKE 2 CIGARETTES. So, you don't like apples? This is often the case for children. Do you know how to get your children to eat fruit? The answer is fruit salad. Do you like fruit salad with yogurt? Make a large bowl of fruit salad regularly from which you can always eat as much as you want. Yes, it is somewhat time consuming to cut everything up—but you have time. It takes the same time to make fruit salad as it does to smoke 2 cigarettes. I've timed it myself. If you didn't smoke 20 cigarettes per day, you would save yourself 100 minutes. And you can eat that fruit salad all day long without becoming fat.

HOT TEA HAS A CALMING EFFECT. Hot drinks give you a nice warm feeling inside. A cup of tea keeps you busy just as long as a cigarette would. Equally important: Tea is associated with cigarettes in the case of very few smokers, in contrast to coffee. And unlike coffee, a hot cup of tea is a classic way to obtain a calming and satisfying feeling. If you find tea is too stimulating in the evening, try Indian chai or herbal teas to avoid the caffeine in standard black or green teas.

ALWAYS EAT UNTIL YOU ARE FULL OR SATISFIED AND NEVER COUNT THE CALORIES! This is dedicated to everyone who has followed too many diets. During the first few months after you quit, never count the calories you are eating—even if it means an extra pound on the scale. Always eat until you feel full. Besides, counting calories is totally passé in modern diets. More about this later. Don´t give your addicted brain a chance to complain and feel frustrated.

At mealtimes, eat until you really feel full—all the more so, if the meal includes meat or fish with lots of salad and other vegetables. But for goodness' sake, I am not saying you should change your eating habits. Just when the opportunity arises—choose steak and salad.

Pasta, cooked until al dente, also enters the bloodstream slowly. This is the reason Italians with a traditional Italian diet (not Italians living in the United States) stay slim. Overcook the pasta and it will turn into a quick carbohydrate. Potatoes, French fries, other potato products, such as chips, and above all highly refined white bread send carbohydrates quicker to the blood than normal sugar. And most Americans have these quick-fattening products every day on their plate. Instead of potatoes, choose vegetables or salad as a side dish. These slow carbs will prevent you from getting fat.

Overall—while dining, give in to the normal feeling of hunger and enjoy your improved sense of taste.

BY THE WAY: DARK CHOCOLATE IS OKAY. Dark chocolate with 70% cacao has quite a lot of calories, about 1,500 in a bar, but in contrast to milk chocolate it contains less sugar. Often, 2 or 3 pieces are enough due to dark chocolate's satisfying intensity of flavor. Chances are, you won't want to eat more and more of it, as is the case with chocolate bars that have a high sugar content. The latter make your blood sugar rise quickly and then drop, and feeling this low sugar level in your bloodstream, you will then devour the rest of the bar.

Constipation When Quitting Smoking

Many have gotten used to it: ciggy, coffee, poop, and the morn-ing digestion is taken care of. Coffee stimulates the digestive system and nicotine has many docking places (receptors) in the vegetative nervous system. Among other things, it causes more movement in the stomach and intestines. Constipation is com-mon during the first 2 weeks after quitting smoking. About 1 in 6 gets it temporarily and it's not a good feeling.

Everyone knows the feeling of relief; ensure that you feel good as quickly as possible. If you are experiencing constipation, you should always eat more fruit and vegetables. Their soluble fiber cleans the intestines. Exercise and drinking more water will also help. Drink 2 to 3 liters a day of water to flush out toxic substances. If all that doesn't work, don't buy laxatives; buy psyl-lium instead in a pharmacy or drugstore. Psyllium is much bet-ter at regulating the activity of the intestines. This is not an eco-tip but is proven by studies. Google "psyllium" at Wikipedia to learn more about it.

One thing is positive: Nicotine causes overproduction of acid in the stomach. Smokers who suffer from heartburn or nervous intestines will soon rejoice over their calmer digestion after quit-ting cigarettes.

Sugar-free Sweeteners

5 cups of coffee per day, each with 2 teaspoons of sugar, amount to 125 calories. Totally unnecessary. That is why no-calorie sweet-eners exist. 2 yogurts that omit sugar save another 60 calories. A large glass of diet cola saves 88 calories. A glass of Coca-Cola contains 11 sugar cubes. With a no-calorie sweetener you can easily save yourself 100 to 200 calories a day, as well as circum-vent the sugar-addiction vicious cycle. Ban normal sugar from

your groceries for a few months. Use only no-calorie sweeteners at home or when you are out and about. Buy drinks, jam, yogurt, pudding, chewing gum, and sweets that contain only sugar-free sweetener. You aren't missing out on anything—you are simply replacing the sugar.

How Healthy Are Artificial Sweeteners?

I am always somewhat touched when smokers who inhale 4,800 toxic substances daily ask me whether no-calorie sweeteners can harm the body. Now, smokers are careful people like everyone else. They put on their seat belts and buy organic fruit in health food shops. So the question is justified. Sugar or sweeteners? The facts:

- Sugar-free sweeteners have no calories and don't make you fat. The agricultural lobby for sugar spreads false information on the Internet that these sweeteners are fattening. This is clearly not the case.
- Artificial sweeteners don´t stimulate insulin release.
- This is the reason that sweeteners don't make you hungry nor do they cause a too low blood sugar level.
- Artificial sweeteners are safe.
- Sugar-free sweeteners provide a dopamine kick by providing a sweet taste without activating the insulin-hunger mechanism (see pages 208–210).

Even the German Nutritional Society (DGE), the equivalent of the RDA, as the leading group of independent experts which constantly evaluates studies and all kinds of nutrients, has a positive view of these products. The DGE certifies that sweeteners are "a good alternative for individuals who wish to reduce weight."[118]

21

Protein—Feeling Full and Happy

Protein Keeps You Slim

You want to keep your current weight? Then you should eat more protein, and especially drink more of it. All modern diets have protein as the key component. *Diet* used to be synonymous with "doing without something," being in a bad mood, and experiencing the yo-yo effect: losing weight but putting it right back on again. In the 1970s, whoever cared about how they looked would have hardly dared enter a restaurant without a caloric table. And then in the 1980s, they probably started counting fat calories and started buying "light" products. The result: unhappy people who were constantly dieting, dissatisfied, and hungry. In the meantime, it's been recognized that diets high in carbohydrates make you hungry. In contrast, protein makes you feel full and happy and maintains the muscle mass, a perfect fat-burning machine. This eliminates the yo-yo effect. So more protein is ideal for you if you want to keep your weight down when you quit smoking.

- Protein sends a signal to the brain that you are full. Being full earlier means you eat fewer calories.
- Protein doesn't stimulate the release of insulin. Thus, you become hungry less quickly and your body can later switch simply to burning fat.
- Protein provides the components to build the neurotransmitter for happiness.
- Protein helps build muscle. Muscles are the protein storage site of the body.
- Muscles burn fat. Lots of it! Each additional kilo (2 pounds) of muscle burns 100 calories additionally daily! Just like that. That's a fact.

Eat more protein. More *lean* meat, more fish, and in between, protein shakes. That shouldn't be too difficult, even for my male readers. First, men prefer eating meat. Second, shakes can be made in just minutes. Vegetarians can use soy protein shakes to remain slim or maintain their weight. But vegetarians rarely have weight problems anyway.

Protein Shakes Reduce Sugar Cravings

When you get the little pangs of hunger or the munchies in the first weeks after quitting smoking, drink a protein shake first instead of eating sweets. Sugary foods will only make you hungrier, fatter, and less satisfied. On the other hand, protein shakes

- give you the feeling of being full
- make it possible to consume fewer calories without feeling hungry
- stimulate the production of happiness transmitter substances
- make you more concentrated, calmer, and less likely to stress out

- speed up the metabolism in general
- taste good and come in many varieties
- are fast and easy to prepare
- can be taken with you wherever you go
- can be consumed at work, between meals

Practical—Just "Shake" Some Protein

What you need: a blender and a drip-proof, lidded cup or thermos for when you are out and about. A handheld blender can also be used but doesn't make the shakes as frothy.

Then, depending on your tastes, fruit (frozen blueberries or raspberries or fresh strawberries, bananas, or oranges); or cocoa powder or coffee, if desired; and natural protein, such as milk, low-fat curd-style cheese, soy, or whey protein. (See the shopping list on pages 225–30.)

A shake can be prepared in the time it takes to smoke a cigarette, no longer than that: In a blender, combine 2 scoops of protein, some water, your choice of fruit, and no-calorie sweetener. Blend for 30 seconds. It's ready in a jiffy. When out and about, you can even use a shaker to prepare your protein drink.

On the Internet site are more recipes for shakes

Protein Tips—Which Type of Protein and How Much?

Milk Protein Shakes

Milk protein keeps you feeling full for a long time. If you are into food rather than milk protein, concentrate then on low-fat curd-style cheese, such as fromage frais, cottage cheese, or farmer cheese, which should be kept in the fridge. The fat content should not be higher than 2%. About a cup of soft cheese contains 24 grams of protein, which is equivalent to that of a 7-ounce steak but with much fewer calories.

Do not prepare just milk- or yogurt-rich shakes, as they contain lots of milk sugar—too many calories and too little protein. Low-fat milk or yogurt should only be used in smaller quanties as a liquid base for shakes made with protein powder. A milk shake without extra protein just doesn´t do anything for you. A protein shake, on the other hand, gives you up to 20 grams of protein per glass.

Soy Protein for Vegetarians

Soy protein concentrate is the first choice for vegetarians. Not everyone likes the taste of soy protein; you either like it or you don't. It tastes a little bit nutty. Strong flavors, such as coffee or chocolate, are the best match for soy protein. Ready-made soy milk has too little protein to make you feel full. Concentrated soy protein, which you can mix yourself, is ideal. Also, when you're out and about, a soy protein shake can make you feel full.

Be on the lookout for deceptive packaging: Some manufacturers mix cheap wheat protein with soy protein. They mark it on the package as: "Contains plant proteins, *usually* soy protein." Check that it contains 100% soy protein. Good sources are health food stores or the Internet.

Milk Protein Powder

To buy milk protein as a concentrate is a waste of money. It is thick, tastes dull, and above all, bloats. Your better bet is to buy a filtered whey protein where most milk sugar is eliminated.

Whey Protein—The Speedy Messenger for the Brain

It really makes sense to buy protein concentrate. "Uhh, a powder . . . ," a lot of people will say. Would you say the same thing about carbohydrate concentrate (flour)? Whey protein is ideal for shakes. The advantages are the following:

- It gets into the bloodstream quickly—much more quickly than milk protein, 3 hours quicker than a piece of roast pork. Whey protein sprints to the brain receptors for happiness, where you have the lack of neurotransmitters as a fresh nonsmoker. So you will be more satisfied and able to concentrate.
- It has almost no fat calories and is rich in calories compared to other high-protein foods, such as meat.
- Whey protein is less expensive than comparable high-protein food. When you calculate the price, ounce for ounce, of whey protein versus protein from other food sources, the concentrated proteins are really less expensive. It only seems more expensive at first glance because you are usually purchasing 30 servings of protein per container.

Do not confuse whey protein with the whey drinks you find in the supermarket. The latter contain little protein but mainly milk sugar, which causes severe bloating.

Where's the best place to buy whey protein? The widest selection can be found on the Internet. Search for "whey protein concentrate," or even better, for high-quality "whey protein isolate." The isolate contains the smallest amount of milk sugar. Leave a container of whey protein at work or carry a ready-made shake in a sealed cup.

Which flavor? If you want to mix the whey protein with cocoa powder, coffee, or fruit, then use vanilla-flavored protein as the basis. This allows you more flexibility in combining it with other flavors. If you mix it on the go in a shaker, just choose your favorite flavor.

Shakes in Place of a Diet

I don´t intend to change your diet. If this were a book on dieting, I would offer you all kinds of recipes from protein-rich lentils to great Asian tofu dishes. But here we are only concerned with keeping your weight in check. And this book should be as practical as possible. Even men and women who would chose death rather than the kitchen and use the stove just to boil water for coffee can use this advice with the greatest of ease.

22

Maintain Your Weight After You Quit Smoking: The Shopping List

From the Internet

When you quit, you should already have everything ready at hand so you don´t put on the extra pounds. Via the Internet you can easily order:

- 1 blender (price: the same as 7 packs of cigarettes, but it will last for years)
- 1 completely watertight drinking cup or thermos. This is for drinking protein shakes when you are on the go (price: one pack of cigarettes)
- 1 (750-gram) container of whey or soy protein, for protein shakes

In the Supermarket

You should buy these products shortly before you stop smoking. With a healthily stocked fridge, you can eat without even thinking about calories. Eat to your heart's content!

- Sugar-free raw ham, cut into extremely thin slices, or chicken if you want something heartier. Both contain little fat and thus few calories.
- Whole wheat bread is better than others. It keeps you feeling full for longer and keeps your insulin level low. But eat it only if you like it! It is not the time to convince yourself to eat something you don´t like.
- 2 or 3 diet frozen meals for when you are feeling really hungry (important: Do not smoke to counter the hunger—eat something!). There are many frozen meals with reduced fat and calories. Choose a brand that has no additives or preservatives, no more than 500 calories for a main course, and tastes great. I cannot repeat it enough: Food should be practical, quickly available, enjoyable, and low in fat and calories. Preparing elaborate dishes while in withdrawal is not anyone's idea of fun. Frozen foods can really make things easier. Eat quickly a full, tasty meal made up of 500 calories, which is better than 100 grams of chips (530 calories) and a bar of chocolate (550 grams). Under no circumstances should you spend an evening feeling hungry. The addicted brain will notice immediately!
- 1 bottle of liquid no-calorie sweetener, or a box of powdered artificial sweetener (you may wish to add a package of single-portion packets of powdered sweetener, for on-the-go).
- 1 package each of frozen raspberries, frozen blueberries, and frozen blackberries. These are cheaper, richer in vitamins, and more practical than buying them fresh. Add 1 package of frozen strawberries, when it is not summer. Frozen berries are ideal for really tasty shakes. Just shake them into your blender without thawing first.

- 10 apples, 10 pears, plus any other kind of fruit, for eating at home or on-the-go, whenever you want and as much as you want. It is important to always have fresh fruit within reach.
- 4 (16-ounce) containers of low-fat yogurt (should have a maximum of 1.5 percent fat).
- 10 (16-ounce) containers of low-fat fromage frais, cottage cheese, or farmer cheese (with no more than 0.5% to 2% fat).
- 4 containers of milk (with 1% to 2% fat), for shakes or use in coffee.
- Various flavors of sugar-free chewing gum
- Diet cola or other sugar-free soft drinks
- Dry red or white wine. If alcohol consumption is part of your lifestyle, then drink wine, not beer. That said, take care that thoughts about wine are not linked to cigarettes.
- Every type of tea, preferably caffeine-free. Try rooibos tea, aromatic herbal teas, or Indian chai. It is always good to have something warm in your stomach.
- 1 package of B vitamin supplements, as well as effervescent magnesium tablets for your nerves. My advice: Take magnesium shortly before going to sleep. This reduces problems in falling asleep, which is part of the withdrawal symptoms.

Things You Shouldn't Buy After Quitting

I believe this list isn't so long. I don't want to disrupt your habits too much. You should always feel full—always! Then you won't even notice that you haven't bought the following products. Maintaining your weight starts in the supermarket. Do not forget your glasses when you go shopping and check the fat and sugar contents of the products you always used to buy. You should never have the feeling that you are going without something. If you cannot live without chocolate pudding with whipped cream, then buy it. There are some other unnecessary pitfalls that you can avoid completely by buying alternatives that are just as tasty.

- **MEAT CONTAINING A LOT OF FAT, SUCH AS PORK OR GROUND MEAT:** Try chicken breast, lean beef, beef tartare, veal, or fish. Going without something is not what this is about, is it? These alternatives contain less fat and fewer calories. Why not spend some of the money you are saving on cigarettes on the somewhat more expensive cuts of meats, which are low in fat, instead of on sausages, pork, or cheap ground meat. Treat yourself to something better.

- **MILK PRODUCTS WITH A FAT CONTENT HIGHER THAN 2%:** Greek yogurt simply has too many calories and fat, without their really adding that much to the taste. If you stir low-fat regular yogurt until it is creamy, it tastes just as good as yogurts with a much higher fat content.

- **MILK PRODUCTS WITH ADDED SUGAR:** For the time being, do not buy these at all. Many milk products, such as yogurt, puddings, and frozen confections, contain sweetener, but you really have to look for them with a magnifying glass on the packaging. The food industry just loves to make you a sugar addict. Instead of buying these, you will knock back so many fruity or chocolate protein shakes with a feeling of lasting fullness that you probably won't even have space in your stomach for any extra desserts and yogurts.

- **COLD CUTS WITH AN EXTREMELY HIGH FAT OR SUGAR CONTENT:** Uncured ham, on the other hand, contains very little fat.

- **SWEETS:** Milk chocolate and other kinds of chocolate bars can contain up to 50% sugar. Change to dark chocolate with 70% cacao content. This keeps your insulin level more stable. Do not store candies in the cupboard at home. You will eat them. If there are none or very few there, you will finally just eat an apple instead. Even when you at first don't feel like it. Finally, you'll be happy just to have something in your mouth for oral satisfaction and it won´t make any difference.

- **SOFT DRINKS CONTAINING SUGAR:** Ouch! These guarantee a hunger attack within 30 minutes. Don't drink them! Many soft drinks now omit sugar, so simply switch products and you aren't really giving up anything!

- **FRUIT JUICES THAT ARE NOT 100% JUICE:** These always contain loads of sugar, often disguised as high-fructose corn syrup. Buy only pure fruit juice and dilute it with carbonated water, like a spritzer, to halve the number of calories.

- **SUGAR:** Replace this completely with no-calorie sweetener both at home and when you are out and about. Here again is the same issue: You are giving up nothing, because you are still experiencing the sweetness!

- **BEER:** Admittedly, this could be a difficult one! But the problem is the following: Beer is usually a smoking cue, closely associated in the brain with lighting up. That makes for a bad start. Also, the quick energy from the beer (malt sugar) is stuffed directly into your fat cells, due to the high excretion of insulin. As your blood sugar level drops quickly below normal, you have to keep topping up. The famous "beer belly" is the classic fat storage result of this. Try wine for a while as an alternative, if alcohol is part of your lifestyle—but only if you feel like it, and if wine is not another cue for lighting up. If you simply cannot do without a beer, then *on no account* should you stop when quitting smoking. Just make sure it's *a* beer, not beers—and really take your time choosing a good beer and savoring it. Avoid lighting up while enjoying your brew.

Okay. Take another look at the list. Was that so terrible? Basically you have only swapped products; you haven't really given up much. An artificial sweetener alone reduces your daily calorie intake by some 100 to 200 calories. *So this is not a diet.*

Eat Out and Lose Weight

Whether you are dining out or eating in the company cafeteria, keep these choices in mind.

- **A STEAKHOUSE IS IDEAL.** Sounds bad? Most men don't find this difficult at all. Don't eat ribs and avoid the French fries or potatoes as sides; choose instead the classic steak and salad combination. You can eat this until you drop.
- **NO HEAVY CREAM SAUCES.** There is certainly grilled fish or roasted meat on the menu, which you won't have to drown in a cream sauce.
- **AVOID DROWNING LEAN PROTEIN MEALS IN KETCHUP.** Ketchup may derive up to one quarter of its calories from sugar, turning a diet-friendly piece of grilled steak into a candy-coated calorie bomb. Use instead a few dashes of spicy hot sauces; use more condiments like pepper or other spices.

- **THAI FOOD AND SUSHI KEEPS YOU SLIM.** Have you ever seen
  overweight Southeast Asians when traveling in Asia? I
  don't mean Asians born in the United States. When
  Asian immigrants over time change their healthy
  traditional diet to a fattening US diet, they become
  obese.[119] Go for Asian food. Thai food and sushi really
  keeps you slim. Indian and other Asian cuisines may
  contain more fat. Go with parboiled rice, not noodles.
  Order steamed or stir-fried dishes and avoid all deep-fried
  dishes and sweet-and-sour dishes that have loads of sugar.

- **IN THE RESTAURANT, TELL THE WAITER WHAT YOU WANT
  FROM THE KITCHEN.** Avoid fatty, creamy sauces. On the
  menu you find pretty much everything with potatoes
  as a side dish. Ask for vegetables instead; have a salad
  as an appetizer or a side dish to your meal. Remember
  you are the guest who is paying. You have no need to
  feel embarrassed.

- **AVOID THE FOLLOWING:**

  - **SIDE DISHES, SUCH AS POTATOES OR MACARONI WITH
    CHEESE:** These drastically increase the blood sugar
    level, making you fat and hungry. Pasta cooked al
    dente and more vegetables are better choices.

  - **DEEP-FRIED FOODS:** Shun these completely. They
    are full of fat. French fries have 3 times as many
    calories as a baked potato, so choose the latter if
    you must have potatoes as a side dish.

  - **BREADED MEAT:** Chicken nuggets or breaded fish
    go right into your spare tire. The bread crumbs
    have loads of fat. Plus, usually these items are
    deep-fried. Eat an alternative if there is one, or
    go somewhere else.

  - **COFFEE:** Always have no-calorie sweetener on you.
    Or choose tea, water, or a diet soft drink instead.

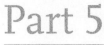

Part 5

The Most Successful Strategies for Quitting

23

How to Become Smoke-*Free*

There is only one thing that makes a dream impossible to achieve: the fear of failure.
—Paulo Coelho

Quitting Is Like Riding a Bicycle

Quitting smoking is like learning to ride a bicycle. In the beginning you have a terrible fear and can think of nothing else but falling off. But if you don't try, and concentrate only on your fear of falling off, you will never learn to ride. Many smokers get caught up in this fear because they have fallen off once or haven't even tried. But when you decide to conquer your fears and land on your face a couple of times and wobble around and get up quickly to give it another try, then you do learn to ride. And once you've learned to, you never need to relearn how to again. This is precisely the same when quitting smoking. Everyone can become a nonsmoker. Down the road it just becomes second nature.

Escaping the Nicotine Trap

You can spend your life fighting the bumpy ups and downs of nicotine withdrawal until your bicycle is in pieces. Or you can decide to change the path.

The fear is greatest when you smoke your last cigarette. But many look forward to the path to freedom and can barely bear to await that day. For the first 2 weeks, the path is not a smooth one until you have overcome the physical addiction barriers and your neurotransmitters have returned to normal. Yet even from the second week, the path begins to get smoother. In the following weeks, there will be some odd bumps caused by conditioning, but you will master these. Perhaps you will lose your balance but you will get back on immediately and continue. These little bumps will become increasingly rare.

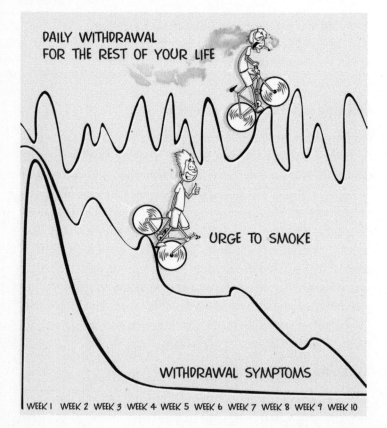

DAILY WITHDRAWAL
FOR THE REST OF YOUR LIFE

URGE TO SMOKE

WITHDRAWAL SYMPTOMS

WEEK 1   WEEK 2   WEEK 3   WEEK 4   WEEK 5   WEEK 6   WEEK 7   WEEK 8   WEEK 9   WEEK 10

Why Doesn't Smoking Less Work?

If you reduce the number of cigarettes, each one you smoke will give you greater satisfaction because it will reduce to a greater degree the tension, irritability, restlessness, and bad mood. These longer periods between cigarettes mean that you will emerge from a much deeper level of nicotine deprivation and in the 7 seconds that the nicotine takes to reach the brain, you will feel a greater sense of relief, enjoyment and well-being than when smoking a cigarette every half hour. At the same time you will be inhaling deeper and more frequently, so that essentially you will be taking in about the same amount of nicotine from the fewer cigarettes. Your obtaining this same amount of nicotine means that there will be little or no reduction of nicotine receptors in the brain. The withdrawal symptoms will remain as intense and will be overcome with fewer but much more satisfying puffs.

Let us say you go down from 15 cigarettes, taking 10 puffs on each, to 10 cigarettes, with 15 deep puffs per cigarette. After 3 months—or 15,000 puffs—you will have learned how extremely valuable to you these last 10 cigarettes have become.

This is not quitting. It is just a new way of remaining dependent. Most smokers who try the reduction method get stuck at a certain number of cigarettes/nicotine inhalations and cannot reduce those any further. They then suffer for years and the feelings of withdrawal between cigarettes become the rule. Life becomes torture and they can only continue with the utmost discipline.

What Works When Quitting Smoking?

The most successful strategy is to quit completely. Set a quitting date and decide on what could provide you with additional support. We know a lot more today than we did 25 years ago when

Allen Carr wrote his first antismoking book. In contrast to these old-fashioned manuals, in which Carr opposes any additional support, the current state of scientific knowledge and the opinion of experts globally recommend quitting with some additional support. I have examined these strategies extremely carefully. With the proper support, you can double or even triple your chances of success. This is not to say, however, that you *must* use additional support! However, total opposition to them, as was the case with this antismoking guru of the 1990s, is wrong from today's perspective. It ignores the fact that smokers differ and that they may need different sorts of support.

Hypnosis, nicotine patches, the drug Chantix, or acupuncture—what helps and what is simply a total waste of money? Do you really need this type of support? And if so, how exactly do you apply it?

Using a technique or product only a little or using it half-heartedly is of little assistance. Make proper use of them or not at all. Otherwise the following happens: "Ah, even nicotine patches didn't help. I'll never manage to quit so I will continue smoking." The incorrect use of therapies or products provides no support in the withdrawal phase. You then blame yourself for failing and become even more convinced that you will always be a smoker.

But everyone can become a nonsmoker. You just have to get back up on that bicycle immediately after you've fallen off, until you've learned to ride properly. The following 4 chapters look at various kinds of help that could provide you with support.

24

Hypnotherapy—Communicating with Your Unconscious

THIS CHAPTER EXAMINES HOW YOU CAN additionally mobilize your unconscious powers against smoking. This you can do through deep relaxation, autosuggestion, or self-hypnosis, but also by means of professional hypnotherapy. For thousands of years, techniques of meditative concentration and restructuring have been used for many purposes. For example, many top athletes use these sources of energy to achieve their goals. Learn how these can be used successfully to support your decision to stop smoking.

Hypnosis Against Addiction

Have you thought of using hypnosis to quit smoking? No? That's a pity, because it is one of the most successful strategies. Hardly any other form of therapy is so successful. A wealth of scientific studies has demonstrated that up to 48% of the participants became nonsmokers within a year.[120] If you compare this to the

7% to 15% success rate with nicotine patches, then you will understand the real power of the unconscious uncovered through hypnosis. But before setting off to search the Internet for a bunch of therapists, first get the lowdown on what clinical hypnotherapy is all about.

In a nutshell: Your addicted brain has not only successfully defeated many years of logic and common sense, but has also overcome your survival instincts that are deeply rooted in the unconscious. No smoker intends to harm him- or herself. Every smoker wants to be healthy, to have a long life, to be free and not to feel compelled to smoke. And yet the nicotine addiction manages to undermine these survival instincts. These desires are "suppressed" deep in the unconscious. If you manage to uncover these unconscious basic needs, then you unleash amazing powers to fight the addiction. But, there is a catch: Accessing your unconscious is not within your own willpower. The powerful unconscious is difficult to reach. Hypnotherapy can open a channel to the unconscious, so you are better in touch with your deep-rooted instincts. Hypnosis is thus a good supplement to this book.

I have provided you with a rational argument of why smoking has no advantages and provides no real enjoyment. Together in this book we have tackled many misconceptions about smoking. If you can also mobilize your unconscious to fight addiction, then you are working at an extremely powerful level. Are you ready to learn more about the unconscious—the most powerful force within you? Then, read on.

The Power of the Unconscious

The human brain has a small conscious memory part and a much larger unconscious memory system. This unconscious memory system determines to a large degree our daily actions without our being aware of this. All our experience and our knowledge are stored in this unconscious memory system. Often this knowledge cannot be expressed in words or accessed. But emotionally we know exactly when we do something right and when we don't, when we deceive ourselves and when we don't. We act and react intuitively most of the time. Each new experience becomes a part of this unconscious knowledge pool and affects our behavior. The biological survival and success programs, which were acquired through evolution, are stored here: the will to survive, breathing (to sustain ourselves with oxygen), and also the urge *not* to harm ourselves. Destructive addictive behavior manages to cloud our will to survive and other unconscious desires, to suppress them and enslave us with obscure fatalistic thoughts, such as, "So what, I have to die of something." See how cunningly addiction undermines our basic instincts. "I could be run over by a bus," you shrug. Of course, you could, but would you deliberately throw yourself in front of a bus? Yet you are smoking yourself to death. You are risking everything, just to inhale lethal substances, because you have become a slave to nicotine. In the case of a heroin addict, this is perfectly clear at first glance. Yet annually only a few thousand die from heroin. *5 million people* die every year as a result of smoking!

Your true instincts have been fogged by the addiction, but these desires can never be completely suppressed. You know that you often deceive yourself, that you do not have a lot of self-confidence in your desire to quit. As long as you smoke, you remain caught in an inextricable smokers' conflict. The worst thing about the addiction is to disregard your own survival instincts, to suppress your desire to quit and put it off for a later time. "Someday I'll stop." This suppression consumes a great deal of your mental energy.

Addiction Is Strong, but Your Unconscious Is Stronger!

In your unconscious, all your aspirations and desires have been stored for a long time, long before you become aware of them much later. You can gain access to these, access to what you've always really wanted. Deep inside yourself you have known for a long time that smoking is not good for you. Possibly you even know that for a long time you have wished to be freer—free to decide without dependence, free of an addiction dictating what and when you have to do something. Deep in your unconscious you want to remain healthy and live for a long time. Nature encoded this in your genetic material: to feel full of energy, to fill each cell with oxygen, with life, to take deep breaths and feel free. Your unconscious knows the way. Your addiction is strong, but your unconscious is much stronger. It knows the true key to your happiness. It has known for a long time that you have had to smoke to avoid withdrawal symptoms but that this really does not satisfy you. The strongest force to fight your addiction is your unconscious wishes. They are an incredible source of power. If you wish, you can rediscover this path.

Access to the Unconscious

Hypnotherapy puts you into a state of trance. This is similar to meditation or deep relaxation and helps open the way to your wishes, which addiction has suppressed. You can also do this yourself by using self-hypnosis and deep relaxation. During this deep relaxation in which disturbing thoughts gradually retreat, you develop a great sensitivity for suggestion and inspiration. In this state, together with your hypnotherapist, you can again uncover and strengthen your suppressed wishes. You must want to and allow it to happen, as it is based on cooperation. Therefore, nothing will happen without your wanting it or letting it happen.

"Okay—but that now sounds very mystical." At first glance, yes, I agree. But the unconscious determines every minute of your life and is at the core of each psychological development. Look at it this way: If you watched a crime story with a cunning police psychologist who creates a profile of the culprit and asks himself why the culprit had to act in this way, then you would have no problem with the fact of accepting the power of the unconscious. Survival instincts in the unconscious possess enormous power. So why not use this for yourself? Uncover this source of power and use it against addiction. There is nothing mystical about that. Hypnotherapy has been successfully tested on smokers under the strictest of scientific conditions.

Stage Hypnosis Is Ineffective

"No way am I going to be a guinea pig." Hypnotherapy or self-hypnosis has absolutely nothing to do with stage hypnosis where apparently hypnotized individuals with no will of their own climb on to a chair or are mesmerized to behave like a rabbit. This is the very reason why so many of us have ambivalent feelings about hypnosis. You fear losing control and being at the mercy of the hypnotist. But nobody who is hypnotized actually does anything against his or her own will. Even before the spectator climbs the stage in a hypnosis show it is perfectly obvious that he or she wants to be the guinea pig. It is part of the game.

"I really would like you to hypnotize away my smoking." Some smokers who come for hypnosis have the expectations of those who consult a stage hypnotist. They feel they are at the mercy of nicotine and now expect the hypnotherapist to mesmerize them in such a strong manner that they never again are able to or want to smoke. They want to put the responsibility on the shoulders of the hypnotist. But hypnotherapy is the total opposite of the orchestrated stage hypnosis. It is not meant to rob you of your willpower but, on the contrary, to mobilize your inner strengths and desires so that you can free yourself from smoking. The most important thing is: You must really want to quit. If, however, you are sent by someone for hypnosis and you do not really want it, the best hypnosis will have no effect.

Milton Erickson Hypnotherapy

"No hypnotist is going to tell me what to do!" You have hit the nail on the head. Authoritarian hypnosis commands do not work, or do so only very briefly only as long as you want to be the "guinea pig." True hypnosis comes from within your own unconscious. And this is precisely where modern hypnotherapy starts. The man behind it was Milton Erickson. Apart from Freud, he is probably one of the most important psychologists of the 20th century. He places individuals in a state of relaxation or trance using very open, vague, and unspecific words. The sentences used during this initiation phase of hypnosis are structured in such a way that you must fill them with your own content and imagine for yourself what certain words mean to you. You do the actual mental work yourself, in a trance state in which you can access the deepest levels of your unconscious mind.

Often stories are told that only you can relate to your own life. That way, suppressed desires are rearranged in the unconscious and brought to the surface. You are getting more in touch with them again. Suggestions made by hypnotherapists are, above all, suggestions that you yourself fill with life. Thus the hypnosis is self-hypnosis. It is the craft of the hypnotherapists to guide the smoker with this open speech pattern and images so that he or she rearranges as much as possible. This requires enormous experience, a particularly intuitive personality, and thorough training. Clinical hypnosis helps to steer a smoker toward a solution in an oriented and therapeutic manner.

"And then what?" The interesting thing is that your behavior becomes increasingly influenced by your unconscious instincts and desires. You find the power to say no to smoking again from a combination of your survival instinct and your feeling that intuitively you are doing the right thing. This is of enormous importance, for in the initial weeks, the addicted brain will use everything possible to fight this process so that you will return to your old ways. Hypnosis fights back by activating inner strengths that run deeper than the addiction.

Hypnotherapy Is Not Mystical

Hypnosis is neither magical nor mystical. The phenomena can be measured and explained. In ECGs—measurement of brain wave activity—hypnotherapy can produce significant changes from short to long waves. For thousands of years now, man has used these changes in the brain waves. Similar long waves can be detected during meditation, yoga, and meditative archery—imagine hitting the bull's eye of not smoking, like an archer aims, and succeeding intuitively. Access to the unconscious areas of the brain is always characterized by these long brain waves. You do it every day—or, rather, every night—when you dream.

"What do dreams have to do with smoking?" Please have a little more patience. Dreams produce an internal balance between what you experienced during the day and your unconscious. Often you will wake up in the morning and know exactly what to do. If you were still confused in the evening, you see things much more clearly in the morning after the creation of this balance. If you have ever meditated, you will know this clear, calm view of things. It is precisely this clear view and this laid-back calm, a certainty of victory, which you need if you want to quit. You must feel that you are doing the right thing and that you will reach your goal regardless of what your addiction whispers to your brain. Both hypnosis and self-hypnosis use this exchange with the unconscious. Try to demystify your connection with the voice of your unconscious, which you have long heard, but which has long—perhaps over decades—been suppressed by smoking.

My advice: Take some time once a day for deep relaxation and self-hypnosis. You will find 4 half-hour self-hypnosis units on the website.

"I don't have the time for things like that. You don't know what my day looks like . . ." You had the time to take time out for all of those cigarettes. A cigarette is 5 minutes of your time. In smoking 20 cigarettes, some 100 minutes of your day have passed. If you have only smoked some of those in your leisure time, then now you would have the time to relax for 10 minutes.

You will have a somewhat restless time in front of you, once you begin to quit smoking and become nicotine deprived. You will notice how much self-hypnosis helps you relax for a moment. Focus like an archer on the most important target in your new life: being free, living longer, and being happy again without nicotine.

The Power of Logic Has Its Limits

In this book I have appealed mainly to the left side of your brain, the logical side that is responsible for willpower. Hypnosis *and* self-hypnosis address the right side in particular. "Even more of this esoteric nonsense," you might say. This, however, can be measured by imaging techniques. Hypnosis activates the right side of the brain while the areas on the left side responsible for willpower and logic are less active.

"And how does that help me?" Precisely! Always think practically. You can try to use your will power to quit or you have the *feeling* deep down inside you that quitting is the only right thing for you. Very different paths appear when your visual, emotional right side of the brain is activated. Solutions are created there that are literally beyond the logical, thinking left side of the brain. Logically, any smoker knows that smoking is damaging and kills in the long term. Smokers are not idiots. Yet many of them do not succeed in quitting. The power of logic has its limits. Logic can make us wake up with a start when we see the negative consequences of smoking. It is an important motivation. Yet the power of unconscious desires and survival mechanisms is stronger. You can circumvent the limitations of your willpower and gain access to your own unconscious through the deep relaxation produced by hypnosis.

The Documented Success of Hypnotherapy

For readers who do not believe in depth psychology and even less in therapists, I will let the figures speak for themselves. Prof. Dirk Revenstorf of the University of Tübingen is a hypnotherapist with the highest international reputation. A hypnotherapeutic program to quit smoking was developed by his faculty. The success rate of this program was 65% after 3 months and 48% after a year.[121] This is amazingly high and has been strictly monitored in scientific studies. The success rate for using nicotine patches after a year is some 7% to 15%, while for behavioral antismoking therapies it is some 20% to 25%. Those who spontaneously decide to go at it alone, for example as a New Year's resolution, without being mentally prepared by reading a book on quitting, have a success rate of 3% to 10% for each attempt. The good news: Several spontaneous attempts can also lead to success and everyone can become a happy nonsmoker.

On account of the high success rate, in 2006 the Scientific Advisory Board of the Chamber of Psychotherapists in Germany recognized that hypnotherapy is an effective means for quitting smoking. So, hypnosis is not some kind of magic trick: Some private health insurance policies even subsidize or assume the full costs of antismoking therapy.

An Overview of Hypnotherapy Studies

"Well, okay, but do precise figures exist on hypnotherapy?" Yes, they do and the numbers speak for themselves. Take a look at how various studies of quitting smoking with the help of hypnotherapy compare.[122] Quite amazing, don't you think?

NUMBER OF PARTICIPANTS	AFTER HOW MANY MONTHS WAS THE NONSMOKING RATE REQUESTED	PERCENTAGE OF SUCCESSFUL NONSMOKERS	DESCRIPTION OF THE HYPNOSIS SESSIONS
615	6 months	44%	1 group hypnosis[123]
48	10 months	50%	1 group hypnosis[124]
48	6 months	50%	5 individual sessions[125]
58	6 months	40% group hypnosis 50% individual hypnosis	3 sessions[126]
75	6 months	45%	1 individual session[127]
30	3 months	60%	1 session[128]

NUMBER OF PARTICIPANTS (continued)	AFTER HOW MANY MONTHS WAS THE NONSMOKING RATE REQUESTED	PERCENTAGE OF SUCCESSFUL NONSMOKERS	DESCRIPTION OF THE HYPNOSIS SESSIONS
37	10–19 months	47% individual hypnosis 36% group hypnosis	1 session[129]
60	12 months	45%	1 session[130]
38	3 months	65%	4 individual sessions[131]
135	7 months	36%	1 group hypnosis[132]
51	12 months	59%	2 individual sessions[133]
106	3 months 12 months	58% 35%	3 sessions[134]

"Why such a complex table?" Using hypnosis over a 12-month period, almost twice as many smokers manage to quit compared to those using behavioral therapy, and even 3 times more quit than did those using nicotine patches. The figures show how important it is to use the power of the unconscious. Hypnotherapy definitely brings results over the long term.

"On the Internet I have read of success rates of 60% to 70% for other methods . . ." That is good advertising! But many other methods are just a scam to rip off smokers. You should always ask, "After how many days or weeks were the smokers consulted: after 3 weeks, 3 months, or after a year?" Pharmaceutical companies also like to use this trick. Only few studies, whether it concerns nicotine patches or other products to help you quit, include data from after 12 months. It is easier to get off with impressive-looking data for 6 months. For this reason remain realistic. Critical inquiry is always good.

Hypnosis FAQS

"HOW DO I FIND THE PROPER HYPNOTHERAPIST?" Hypnosis is often offered by amateurs, with little or no training. Unfortunately, you will find many such scams on the Internet. In any case, check the qualifications of the hypnotherapists. Hypnotherapy is a sophisticated process that should only be offered by psychotherapists and qualified professionals who have undergone demanding further training as hypnotherapists. It is a good sign if they have completed training at a recognized hypnosis association, such as MEG (Milton Erickson Society for Clinical Hypnosis).

"WHAT IS A TRANCE, REALLY?" We all know the everyday trance when we are deeply immersed in something and forget everything else around us. Trance is quite similar to meditation or deep relaxation. You can stop this deep relaxation state at any time and are not dependent on a hypnotist's clicking his fingers. In the trance, you hear everything that is said and you feel totally real in both time and location. "What is the use of a trance?" During the trance, the hypnotherapist can communicate with the unconscious part of your brain without interference from your reasoning or your addicted memory.

"I PROBABLY CANNOT BE HYPNOTIZED. CAN EVERYBODY BE HYPNO-TIZED?" Most people can adopt a trance state if they feel involved and have trust. This can be practiced in the same way as meditation or autogenic training is learned. The speed and the depth of the trance differ between individuals. For quitting smoking, a medium depth of trance is sufficient.

The Hypnosis Program

I have worked for the last 10 years as a nonsmoking coach with hypnotherapy to help smokers of all ages quit. I am using the Milton Erickson method of hypnotherapy that has proven in studies and in my own experience to be highly successful. This is the reason that I wanted to make it available also for this non-smoking program as an addition at the lowest possible cost. On the homepage you can download it:

251

- 4 nonsmoker hypnosis sessions, 25 minutes each, which help you to *become* and *remain* smoke-free
- 2 hypnosis sessions that accompany you *before* quitting and 2 in the phase *after* you quit

Why 4 Different Hypnosis Parts?

Before quitting, smokers are torn between whether they will manage to quit this time, whether they will "miss" something, or whether "now" is the right time to quit. Hypnosis makes you more focused before quitting and mobilizes the deep feeling of truly doing what is right for yourself.

After quitting, the addicted brain wants to make itself heard every day. Most books and nonsmoking programs leave you alone after you quit. But it is really here that smokers need the most support. Hypnosis reduces the stress in the first weeks by gaining strength and serenity from your unconscious.

THE BOTTOM LINE

- ▸ Addiction superimposes itself on the natural survival instincts and desire for health. These are suppressed in the unconscious.
- ▸ It is important to uncover these unconscious survival instincts again when you quit smoking and to use the enormous power of your unconscious against addiction.
- ▸ One cannot access the unconscious by using one's willpower.

- ▶ Deep relaxation, auto-suggestion, self-hypnosis, and hypnotherapy grant access to this unconscious source of power and mobilize it.
- ▶ The longer brain waves, which open access to the unconscious, have been used by various disciplines for thousands of years to focus on the essential.
- ▶ The techniques that tap into the right side of the brain to gain access to the unconscious powers are an ideal complement to the conscious, left-brain, active knowledge offered in this book.
- ▶ Hypnotherapy, as a professional supplement, is one of the most successful methods for quitting smoking.

NOTE: If you do not want additional support such as nicotine patches, you can skip the next 3 chapters and continue reading on page 276, "The Last Cigarette." For smokers who are strongly addicted or those who usually give up after the first few days, the following additional support could be important.

25

Nicotine Replacement Therapy—An Aid or a Business?

FAQs About Nicotine Patches

CAN YOU BECOME ADDICTED TO NICOTINE PATCHES? The chances of becoming addicted to patches are practically zero.[135] The quick fix from a cigarette is missing. Nicotine patches slowly and permanently raise the level of nicotine in the blood.

WHY DOES IT WORK TO REDUCE NICOTINE WITH PATCHES BUT NOT WITH SMOKING FEWER CIGARETTES? When you smoke less, you suffer more from the ups and downs of the nicotine level in your blood. The less you smoke, the more precious each cigarette becomes, because the feeling of relief from your withdrawal symptoms (which you rationalize as enjoyment) when you finally smoke appears to be greater. With patches, the attempt is made to systematically wean the nervous system off nicotine by maintaining a constant reduction of stable nicotine level in the blood, as it is the fluctuations that cause you to smoke at set intervals to relieve tension, irritability, and restlessness. Therefore, it is important to maintain this constant nicotine replacement for several weeks and to taper off it quite slowly, subtly, and systematically.

254

DO YOU REALLY NEED TO USE NICOTINE PATCHES? No, far too often smokers are talked into believing that the withdrawal systems are unbearable and that they will not manage without nicotine patches. Both are wrong. The first part of this chapter will discuss these issues further.

WHEN ARE NICOTINE PATCHES WORTHWHILE? If you are a heavily addicted smoker or have frequently admitted defeat in the first week, a softer transition could improve your chances. This only works when you use the product correctly. The second part of this chapter will examine this.

Part 1 Making a Business of Fear

The combination of creating a fear of failing and a fear of purported bad or lifelong withdrawal symptoms makes for good business. The pharmaceutical industry is all too keen to offer nicotine replacement products for those wishing to quit. The proud sum of 1.7 billion is spent annually on such products. But what really lies behind this making a business out of fear?

FEAR OF NOT SUCCEEDING: Before you, millions of people have succeeded without nicotine patches. Listen: As a smoker, do not let others belittle your ability to quit independently. 8 out of 10 smokers manage to quit (see page xiii). And 90% of them do it without any external help. The pharmaceutical industry simply ignores this massive number of successful ex-smokers. Instead, it publishes allegedly low success rates of smokers who have "failed" without the help of pharmaceutical products. That is a lie, precisely because ex-smokers are enormously successful at quitting. These ex-smokers—not the pharmaceutical companies—are some of the best sources for the most effective strategies for quitting.

FEAR OF WITHDRAWAL SYMPTOMS: The pharmaceutical industry, as well as many doctors, exaggerates withdrawal symptoms unnecessarily. In fact, the physical symptoms disappear after 4 to 5 days. Most smokers can cope amazingly well with the physical withdrawal symptoms for a few days, especially when they know it is only for a few days! The decisive question is: For the rest of your life, do you want to feel these little twinges of withdrawal symptoms every day, or do you want to get rid of them once and for all?

FEAR OF NEVER BEING ABLE TO ENJOY LIFE AGAIN: This is an unjustified fear. Nicotine will vanish completely from your system after 4 days, and after 3 weeks, the neurotransmitter system in your brain will have recovered. You will enjoy life fully as soon as your brain is no longer urging you to smoke. Look at it this way: An interesting experience lies before you. Feel the positive changes in your body as it frees itself daily more and more from the addiction and the toxins. You already know you will feel better as a nonaddict. ("No, I do not know that at all." Then you have skipped chapter 11. Please do read this chapter.)

FEAR OF CONSTANTLY MISSING CIGARETTES: Many more smokers fail in quitting on account of psychological and emotional dependence than from physical symptoms. The reason is the following: Smoking is still regarded as advantageous, as stress reducing, and as relaxing. This creates the illusion of doing without something. And this cannot be "patched" by smokers. But you know better: Enjoyment is nothing more than nicotine dependence. Smoking has no psychological advantages. On the contrary; it makes you nervous, restless, and moody, and places you under stress. The logical consequence: You will feel better without cigarettes. You are giving up nothing. You stand only to gain.

Patching Over Is Not Enough

The mind is decisive in quitting smoking and for this reason nicotine replacement products are overestimated if you do not work on your belief-system as well. A doctor who prescribes only nicotine patches for patients is someone who forces them to jump from a 3-meter springboard while knowing that they cannot swim. They will experience panic and fear of what is going to ensue. You really have to see through the nicotine trap beforehand and understand that you will feel better in the absence of cigarettes. "Patching things over" is rarely successful, because the patches do not address smokers' powerful emotional attachments to the act of smoking.

However, nicotine replacement products can be useful for heavy smokers in combination with other components (for example, this antismoking program) and for smokers who want to have it "a little easier." But it is fatal if this "having it a little easier" already conceals the doubt that you will succeed. When the brainwashing about enjoyment and the alleged advantages of cigarettes has been overcome, then you will not fall for the temptation to smoke again.

Already Failed with Nicotine Patches? No Problem!

"Well, I have already tried nicotine patches and even then I didn't manage. I really am a hopeless case." No, you are not. You are in the best of company, for wrongly used nicotine patches help no one. And now you will discover why you are not a failure just because you didn't manage with nicotine patches.

In medical studies, a meager 15% of smokers manage to quit using nicotine patches. In real life, when smokers buy and apply the patches themselves, the success rate is much lower, around 7%.[136] This corresponds to the success rate of those who spontaneously decide to quit smoking.[137] 5% to 10% of smokers who quit spontaneously without help succeed each time they try (depending on the study cited). Patches have had little positive effect on the success rate.

The brochure of a nicotine patch manufacturer even maintains that only 3% manage to quit without help. This strategy is meant to talk the smokers into believing that without nicotine patches, it is almost impossible to kick cigarettes. But what counts as an attempt to stop in this context? The facts are the following: Most smokers make several attempts at quitting, and 8 out of 10 will succeed! Even more interesting: In an analytical overview of 90 nicotine replacement studies that was sponsored by the pharmaceutical industry, a "significant" effect of nicotine replacements was reported. In studies not sponsored by the industry, this was only true in a quarter of the cases, and even there, success was described as "moderate" or "modest."[138]

So, did you fail? No, you probably

- had too high expectations that you would succeed by using only nicotine patches
- applied the patch too low and for too short a period of time
- knew too little about the nicotine trap and in the back of your mind still believed in the benefits of smoking

"But surely, you must be more successful using nicotine patches?" If that were so, then the number of smokers in the population would have dropped dramatically since the introduction of nicotine replacement products in the 1990s. However, the rate of quitting has not increased compared to the 30-year period between 1960 and 1990; that is, the period prior to the invention of the nicotine patch. After the first official warnings of lung cancer in the United States in the 1960s, the age of male smokers went down more than 30% until 1990. Nothing but success-ful ex-smokers, without nicotine replacement products.

258

The Business of Keeping You Hooked

"But surely patches take away the horrible withdrawal symp-toms." Smokers are being regarded increasingly as medical cases that cannot be asked to tolerate "the severe" withdrawal symptoms when quitting on their own. *Never let anyone try to tell you that you can't make it on your own.* Physical dependence on nicotine is very low. In contrast to opium or heroin, the symp-toms of nicotine withdrawal are minimal and very short-lived.

Are you aware of the connection between the cigarette indus-try and the sale of nicotine patches? The cigarette manufacturers keep trying to make us think that it is difficult to quit. The more talk there is of fear of withdrawal and failing, the better they can control their customers. And so, by now, tobacco companies have invested heavily in the manufacture of nicotine replace-ment products! At first glance, there would seem to be no logic to this. In actual fact, however, while seeming to advocate this method of stopping smoking, the industry can constantly publi-cize how difficult it is to kick nicotine. And as 93% of smokers "fail" when using self-applied nicotine replacement products, it is one great business to be in: Spread the fear of quitting and frustrate those who are willing to quit with stories of failure. A small detail is a great example of this linking of the cigarette industry and the pharmaceutical industry: On the packaging of certain nicotine replacement products, as little advice as possible is given on quitting.[139] More knowledge would unnecessarily increase the success rate. The financial investment of the wealthy tobacco industry is relatively small. And the shortfall in turnover from quitting cigarettes is compensated for by the increased turnover in nicotine replacement products. What a fantastic business model.

Your Decision Is Your Success

More numbers, because they don't lie: Successful ex-smokers—
90%—have managed to quit and have shown that they have the
ability to cope with withdrawal symptoms for a few days. Yet pharmaceutical studies of smokers adopt a very different perspective
and distort this success. Of 511 studies published on quitting smoking, 91% were about pharmaceutical aids and only 9% showed
which factors were important for smokers if they didn't use these
"aids."[140] You could learn so much more from those successful
ex-smokers and their strategies, than by listening to the manufacturers that hope you'll fail and go back to smoking. My advice:
Surround yourself with successful ex-smokers and really make
use of their help when quitting. Which ex-smokers do you know?
Who could you ask tomorrow to be your "buddy" when you quit?
Ex-smokers like to help because they know what it is all about.

Your decision to smoke the last dirty cigarette is the most
important one. What you need to do first is to

- rid yourself of the brainwashing about the alleged
  benefits of smoking
- understand the disadvantages of smoking for your mood,
  energy, concentration, and ability to cope with stress
- classify "withdrawal symptoms" time-wise: nicotine
  withdrawal (3–4 days), resetting of the neurotransmitter system (3 weeks), then the overcoming of social
  and other conditioning (1–2 months)
- clarify in your own mind that you no longer want to
  cheat yourself

This way this short time and the path to freedom will be easier. Do not let others make you believe anything and do not let
yourself be belittled and think that you cannot manage to stop
without additional aids.

Part 2 How to Benefit from Nicotine Replacement Products

Now we come to the positive aspects of nicotine replacement products. Some of them are supposed to make life more pleasant, like lettuce that has been already washed and chopped, or ready-made meals. The lettuce loses its vitamins through over-handling and the ready-made meal is packed with additives, but they are both really nice and practical. Nicotine replacement products are among these convenience products. Most of you won´t need them, for you have seen through the nicotine trap. However, should you wish to take nicotine replacement products, then keep in mind that you are using them only to make things a bit more pleasant and not because you would otherwise not manage to quit. There is a major difference. Quitting smoking is not a competition to see who can withstand the most misery. Only success counts. I know only too well the anxieties and fears that come with contemplating the first day without a cigarette. In panic, one would prefer to "patch it over"—"Give me anything that will help." But many smokers do not fail to quit because of the nicotine withdrawal in the first days; actually, they backslide later, because they continue to believe that smoking is a benefit and an enjoyment that they now "have to go without."

Nicotine Patches for Heavy Smokers

Severely addicted smokers can benefit from nicotine patches as they are more prone to the withdrawal symptoms and especially to the mood swings. You can discover your degree of addiction by taking the Fagerström tests (see pages 55–56).

Even smokers who, in spite of knowing everything about quitting, simply do not believe in themselves or have major fear of withdrawal or have failed frequently in the past can be helped by nicotine patches. But have you noted now what smoking has done to your self-confidence? Yet another reason to liberate yourself.

"I am not a heavy smoker but I have nothing against a little help. I could put on a few patches." Please don't. Do it correctly. The reason that only 7% manage to quit by nicotine patches is their wrong application. The most prevalent errors are using them for too short a time and using too low a dose. Smokers take ages to decide to quit, but they want to be rid of nicotine replacement products as quickly as possible. Give yourself 8 to 12 weeks. That also gives you the chance to practice coping with many situations without cigarettes. Then nicotine replacement products increase the success rate by 50% to 70%. A compilation (meta-analysis) of 111 studies shows this.[141]

"Why now 50% to 70%? And, what do chances of success mean, anyway?" Many people use a number of components. An example: If smoker seminars can produce some 20% of non-smokers after one year, then, in combination with the correctly applied patches, the chances of success increase by some 35%. That is a very different story compared to the meager 7% of smokers who tried simply to "patch over" smoking.

The better prepared you are, the higher the chances of success. Use the 30-day Internet program (www.my30dayquitsmokingcoach.com), read the book carefully, use the self-hypnosis downloads from the homepage, and possibly take nicotine replacement products or the drug Chantix (see next chapter). Quitting has a lot less to do with willpower and a lot more with preparation, knowledge, and with strategies to avoid relapse.

So, Who Should Take What?

Here are the recommendations of the industry producing nicotine replacements.

NUMBER OF FAGERSTRÖM POINTS*	RECOMMENDED NICOTINE REPLACEMENTS[142]
1–2	Nicotine chewing gum or lozenges
3	1 patch
4–7	1 patch plus 6–12 pieces of chewing gum or lozenges, as required

*see pages 55–56

I doubt that smokers with a low dependency of 1 to 2 points in the Fagerström test really need nicotine chewing gum and that this has any added value. In the case of social smokers with a low physical dependency, the main point is to unlearn the conditioned smoking triggers. Whoever uses nicotine gums in these situations only shows that he or she has not understood the nicotine trap.

Application Advice

- The combination of patches plus chewing gum or lozenges is the most successful. Up to one quarter of smokers are still nonsmokers 12 months later.[143]
- Use nicotine patches for long-term treatment for a constant blood nicotine level. Take chewing gum or lozenges only as an exception, in the case of an addiction attack. Do not simply chew or suck nicotine to feel better or whenever you suspect that you could feel withdrawal, otherwise you will take in too much nicotine. You must keep the precise daily chewing gum balance in your head and taper off the chewing gum over time. It is best to keep notes.
- The more cigarettes you have smoked in the past, the higher the dosage should be.

- 1 cigarette contains approximately 1 mg of nicotine. 20 cigarettes would be equal to a patch that releases 20 mg.
- Under no circumstances should you smoke while using the patches! Otherwise you may consume more nicotine than usual. Apart from that, if you smoke you have not really made the decision to quit.

Correct Dosage

Again, using too low a dose and for too short a time are the main mistakes made with nicotine replacement products. You need to have a precise and planned approach.

You should follow the calculated and selected nicotine dosage for at least 2 weeks. Officially, 3 to 4 weeks are recommended. Following that, you change to the next lower level of nicotine patch. The advantage of prolonged application: Smoking behavior is uncoupled from the learned daily situations. You are gradually overcoming the conditioning.

After a mini-test I did, where I was wrongly advised in 5 out of 10 pharmacies, I decided to include the dosage in this book. All suppliers offer 3 levels of patches: low (about 7 mg), medium (about 14 mg), and high (about 20 mg). Always pay attention to the suggested dosage of "release of nicotine" on the packaging.

- **IF YOU SMOKE 15 TO 20 CIGARETTES DAILY:** You need medium strength.
- **IF YOU SMOKE MORE THAN 20 CIGARETTES DAILY:** You should start with the patch with the highest level of nicotine.
- **IF YOU SMOKE 40 CIGARETTES DAILY:** You will require 2 patches with the highest level of nicotine.
- **IF YOU SMOKE LESS THAN 10 CIGARETTES DAILY:** Then take only nicotine chewing gum without additional

patches. The chewing gum is suitable for social and very light smokers.[144] But to stay honest, make a definite decision. As a social or light smoker, you must never smoke again. Tell yourself again and again that smoking has no benefits for you. I doubt if very light smokers even need nicotine chewing gum, if their resolve to quit remains firm.

Only Use Nicotine Chewing Gum During the Period of Physical Withdrawal

"I have not smoked for 4 months but chew nicotine chewing gum now and again." That is nonsense. Your body has long become free of the addiction. Why give your body nicotine it does not need? In this phase, your main concerns are the psychological aspects, and for this reason you should learn to escape the conditioning that triggers smoking. The craving for a cigarette becomes rarer as time passes and it only lasts for a few minutes. Chewing nicotine gum will be of no benefit to you. The body no longer craves it.

No Deals—Stop Smoking!

About one fifth of those who use nicotine patches use them to bump up their nicotine addiction instead of wean themselves off it. 3 examples:

"I smoke less and apply additional patches." Forget this strategy as you will only become more dependent on nicotine between the patches and continuing to smoke.

"Well, I smoke a few just as a reward and then chew nicotine gums. That's my compromise for health." My opinion: This will never work.

"I will use nicotine patches to stop smoking for a while

because they are less damaging." Taking a break from smoking is not a real decision to get rid of the addiction but simply a bad deal. In this way the addiction prevails; you are getting your fix via the patches instead of cigarettes. So make a definite decision and make use of replacement products, if required, without going back to smoking. "Quitting for a little while" simply does not work.

So now you've made your decision. Look forward to your new life without cigarettes, using nicotine patches, if at all, only as a brief aid toward achieving your goal.

THE BOTTOM LINE

- ▶ Smokers who have not managed to quit in the past using nicotine replacement products are not losers but had too high, false expectations of this form of therapy.
- ▶ The mind remains the major factor for success. Millions of smokers have proven this.
- ▶ Smokers who use a nicotine patch dosage that is too low or for too short a period of time have little more chance of success than do those who spontaneously decide to quit smoking without any help.
- ▶ The correct use and the combination of nicotine patches and chewing gum in contrast raise the chances of success significantly.
- ▶ Above all, smokers who have a strong addiction can systematically taper nicotine intake through the use of nicotine replacements.
- ▶ Nicotine replacement should only be used in the period of physical withdrawal and not longer in the phase of learning to cope with the conditioning of smoking triggers.

⚠️ **WARNING:** Keep nicotine patches out of the reach of children and animals.

266

DISCLAIMER:

Only *you* and an experienced doctor of your choice can decide whether you want to use nicotine replacement products. Medical advice can only be given by a doctor who has a chance to personally observe and understand your health condition and objective. The information given in this book is solely intended for information purposes and should not be taken for medical advice. The author and the publisher disclaim all responsibility for all liabilities, loss, or risk, personal or otherwise, which is incurred as a consequence, directly or indirectly, of the use and application of nicotine replacement products or for readers who ignore the warnings printed on nicotine replacement products. By virtue of this Disclaimer you may not hold us responsible for any adverse effect you suffer from these products and you may not look to us to indemnify you from your own decision to use these products.

26

Acupuncture— Faith Doesn't Move Mountains

THE INTERNET IS FULL OF OFFERS for acupuncture to help quit smoking. Many alternative practitioners and doctors also want to earn something from alternative-oriented smokers who are suffering. Acupuncture points that have a relaxing effect are selected and stimulated either manually or electronically. Sometimes the acupuncturist uses a soft laser without needles, so as to cater to the target group of points that is sensitive to pain. Also, needles that stay in the ear for a week for "better effect" are used. So far, so good.

Therapists love to talk of their success statistics even when not a single smoker is interviewed after 12 months. Of course, there are cases where acupuncture has helped people to quit smoking. But would these smokers possibly have succeeded in quitting smoking without acupuncture? Let us examine this in greater detail. Perhaps somewhere in the back of your head, you have thought of acupuncture as a means of support. That is exactly why, before running off and investing money in acupuncture, it is worth taking a look at the proven success rates in studies. How do smokers who have quit by using acupuncture compare to those who have managed it without help? At any rate, faith in the needles can move mountains. For this reason, studies divide smokers into 2 groups. One group undergoes proper acupuncture treatment and the others are "just treated with needles" where no acupuncture points exist. The results are not very convincing: in an overall analysis of 24 studies, the number of smokers who had received acupuncture and were ex-smokers after 12 months was no different than in the case of smokers who had "needles simply placed anywhere."[145] The alleged addiction points did not seem to yield results. Faith doesn't move mountains. When you hear of smokers or know smokers who quit by using acupuncture, that is certainly true. But these are perhaps smokers who would have quit anyway.

27

Chantix—Reconquering the Receptors That Make You Happy

IMAGINE THAT NICOTINE COULD REACH THE brain, only to find its receptors were already occupied. After a short time, you'd simply have no desire to smoke because you would not be able to experience the kick you get from nicotine. At the same time, at the occupied receptors, some release of neurotransmitters would need to stimulate the receptors that would cause you to feel fewer withdrawal symptoms. Research went into this very mechanism for many years. The substance in the medication Chantix, which is available on prescription, does exactly this: It occupies the receptors, blocking them from nicotine, and stimulates enough transmitters to reduce withdrawal symptoms and the urge to smoke. As a result, smoking offers little satisfaction, making it easier to quit.

3 Times More Nonsmokers with the Help of Chantix

Medications may help to relieve withdrawal symptoms. Chantix increases your chances of success of becoming smoke-free particularly during the first weeks after quitting, when the pressure to smoke is at its highest. But the media celebrated Chantix as a lifestyle pill, exaggerating its success, and giving the impression that taking a pill is all there is to it. This created totally false expectations. In fact, only 35% of smokers manage to remain nonsmokers after 6 months of taking Chantix, and 23% after a year of doing so. Therefore, with the help of Chantix, the chances of going from smoker to nonsmoker are 3 times higher than of going at it alone with just a New Year's resolution, at which only 5% to 7% of the smokers succeed. Chantix is by no means a miracle drug. It is a serious drug, and can have serious side effects. *Only a doctor who prescribes it and closely monitors side effects can take the responsibility for your use of Chantix.*

Chantix was tested in some studies without intensive consultation, more or less with the idea, "Let's see who manages to quit just with this pill." Additional consultation would have made it unclear how successful Chantix really is in supporting smokers to quit, versus what other factors are really at play. The chances of success increase significantly, however, when it is additionally supported with intensive consultation and self-assessment of one's smoking behavior.

Become and Remain a Nonsmoker

Many smokers start smoking again between 3 and 6 months after quitting, although they have long since become nonsmokers.

 IMPORTANT: Chantix may help you become a nonsmoker but not to remain a nonsmoker!

Why do so many go back to smoking? Some ex-smokers continue to secretly believe in the benefits of smoking and think they could become occasional smokers. This will never work. Consider, for example, the story of Monika:

> I had once stopped for 6 months. Then I tried a cigarette simply to see what it would feel like and I did not have the feeling that the cigarette was satisfying the way it had been in the past. It was nothing special. In fact, it was rather horrible. I had to smoke several until I could enjoy smoking again.

What really happened here? Firstly, Monika describes how insignificant the effect of a cigarette became when she had become a nonsmoker (once her neurotransmitters had returned to normal). Then she also describes how she had to smoke several cigarettes to feel the enjoyment of a cigarette. In other words, she had to smoke to become addicted again and change the neurotransmitters to feel enjoyment and to "be able to" free herself of the withdrawal symptoms again by smoking. Monika is entirely unaware of this mechanism. Look at how she turns the issue to reformulate it as a benefit. "I had to smoke several until I could enjoy smoking again." Even a second Chantix therapy would not help Monika because she's not understood the nicotine trap. The story of starting to smoke again is almost always told like this: ". . . and then I tried one again. It tasted horrible. I am such an idiot to be a smoker again."

When you become a non-smoker, never try another cigarette!

How Does Chantix Compare with Other Antismoking Strategies?

CHANTIX VERSUS BEHAVIORAL THERAPY: The success of Chantix is about equivalent to that of behavioral therapies and antismoking courses without medication.

CHANTIX PLUS BEHAVIORAL THERAPIES: A combination of various components may yield better results. Working on your mind and analyzing your smoking behavior, *plus* additional support in the initial phase to reduce withdrawal symptoms, may be optimal. Here, Chantix may double the success rate of behavioral therapy! Only 5% of smokers combine both components. One thing is very apparent: Mental preparation is also the key to success here.

CHANTIX VERSUS A PLACEBO (A PILL WITHOUT AN ACTIVE SUBSTANCE): In the first 3 months, 44% of the study participants who were on Chantix had become nonsmokers compared to 18% of those taking a placebo.[146] After almost a year, 23% of those on Chantix were still nonsmokers compared to 8% of those taking a placebo. Almost 3 times as many smokers managed to become nonsmokers through blockage of the receptors. And they remained nonsmokers.

After a few months of being a nonsmoker, read the chapters on smoking and the mind again and fill out again the questionnaires in the learning program on the website, to see how much better you are. And help other smokers quit as well. This refreshes the memory of what it felt like when you were still addicted.

CHANTIX VERSUS NICOTINE PATCHES: In such comparative studies, it is important that both groups are similar. Otherwise you end up comparing apples and oranges. Perhaps the participants in the various groups smoked more or were more dependent or . . . The devil lies in the details. The study participants were divided into groups in such a way that on average, the number of cigarettes smoked, the number of attempts to quit, the grade of addiction, the length of time of being a smoker, the proportion of men and women, and age groups were comparable.[147] After a year, 1 in 4 using Chantix and 1 in 5 using nicotine patches were nonsmokers. Chantix showed a higher success rate than nicotine patches did. In the Chantix group, the occurrence of yearning for cigarettes (craving) was rarer, as were such withdrawal symptoms as the desire to inhale into the lungs, restlessness, irritability, and negative feelings.

CHANTIX VERSUS ZYBAN: Zyban is another approved medication for those wishing to quit smoking. You will find it on many Internet sites, as it is more successful than nicotine patches but has many more side effects. In spite of this, direct comparisons have been made between Chantix and Zyban. Here are the figures to round off the picture: After a year, 23% of those on Chantix, 15% of those on Zyban, and 10% of those on a placebo were still nonsmokers.[148]

Nicotine patches may double and Chantix may triple the chances of becoming a nonsmoker.[149] You will have also added to your chances of success—no matter how you decide to quit—if you are more than well prepared and know that smoking is of no benefit to the mind.

Possible Side Effects

The most common side effects of Chantix are headaches, sleep disturbances, strange dreams, and nausea. Studies show that some 11% of smokers taking Chantix stop the therapy on account of the undesirable side effects.

⚠️ **WARNING:** Whoever tries to quit smoking can succumb to temporary depression. An experienced doctor explains to patients that they should stop taking Chantix immediately should severe depression or noticeably alarming changes in behavior occur, and contact the doctor immediately. Anyone suffering from or who has suffered from a psychiatric illness or severe depression should definitely not take Chantix![150]

Individual cases have been documented showing signs of severe depression and agitation, and suicides on Chantix have also been documented. There have been quite extensive negative press reports. In 2009, the European Medicines Agency (EMA) carried out careful tests with particular attention to suicide and depressive illnesses in cases where Chantix had been prescribed. No causal relationship could be identified (as of March 2011). However, this result may or may not hold true for the future and many Chantix studies were industry funded, which may have created a conflict of interest. It is your and your doctor's obligation to find out the current opinion and treatment guidelines in your country of residence.

THE BOTTOM LINE

- ▶ Chantix occupies the receptors for nicotine in the brain. In this way the yearning for cigarettes, the withdrawal symptoms, and the satisfaction of smoking are reduced.

- ▶ Chantix may triple the chances of *becoming* a nonsmoker. *Remaining* a nonsmoker depends on you and how well you have recognized the nicotine trap.

- ▶ Advice, prescription, and therapy monitoring from an experienced doctor are obligatory, as the medication must be stopped immediately in the case of such side effects as depression or mood swings.

28

The Last Cigarette

Before You Quit

- ❏ Have you made a list of what you don't like about smoking and why you no longer wish to smoke? (Page 181)
- ❏ Have you analyzed when you smoke and which triggers make you smoke? (see page 129)
- ❏ Have you looked at the first 10 days of the Internet program?
- ❏ Have you picked a friend as a coach and helper? That is really important.
- ❏ Did you decide if you want to use nicotine replacement products or other medications as support?
- ❏ Have you bought magnesium and B vitamins to support your nervous system?
- ❏ Did you fill your fridge with the right food, proteins, and sweeteners from the shopping list (see pages 225–30)?

You want to avoid staying in the addiction cycle due to sweets and to prevent putting on weight.

This Is Not How You Quit

Simply sticking on a few patches without understanding what smoking does to your mind is like jumping from a 3-meter springboard without being able to swim. For this reason, only 5% to 6% of those who are unprepared succeed to paddle over to the edge of the nonsmoking pool and are of course frustrated. But you are now well prepared. You know exactly how nicotine addiction works. You won't drown in the pool because you no longer talk yourself into believing that nicotine makes you able to concentrate better, improves your mood, and reduces stress. You no longer belittle the consequences of smoking. You know that the period when things are more stormy is limited to 2 weeks and that the waters will calm again the more consistently you show your conditioned brain who is the boss. You decide your own life. You also know that nonsmokers are no less happy than smokers and that ex-smokers feel more stable and fit without nicotine. You know what you want: Nothing less than your freedom. You have everything that you need to succeed. Now all you have to do is jump. Don't be afraid of the cold water. You can swim. Jump! Today!

Bear Witness to Your Last Cigarette

Smoking your last cigarette is a dramatic moment. The faces of smokers in my seminars always show a mixture of panic, fear, and nervous expectation. Excitement and fear of freedom.

Smoke that last cigarette in front of a mirror. Watch yourself very carefully. Concentrate on how the carcinogenic toxic substances enter your lungs and fill them with poison. Be happy that you are getting rid of this tyrant. Only you decide in the future. It is your life. Delight in breathing freely again. Take pleasure in your new life!

After the Last Cigarette

Throw all your smoking utensils away. Put them in the trash bin outside your home:

- ashtrays, lighters, matches
- cigarettes and every other form of tobacco

Brush the last toxic substances from your teeth.

If you feel like it, take the car for cleaning inside, bring the curtains to the cleaners, and sweep the last of the poison out of your apartment.

And today, only do things you take pleasure in. Distract yourself. Like a marathon runner, think only in stages. You only have to remain smoke-free today. Tomorrow is another stage. And each stage—in contrast to the marathon—will get easier.

29

Strategies to Avoid Slips and Lapses

The Camera from Above

Many smokers, particularly heavy smokers, manage to successfully overcome the physical withdrawal more gently with nicotine patches or medication. Once they have this phase behind them, they are fairly amazed at the appearance of conditioned smoking triggers and that these can cause such a strong craving for a cigarette. Do you remember chapter 11? For me, it is a key chapter. And because one cannot fully recall it often enough, here is the core message again: Through neurotransmitters, nicotine unnecessarily conditions many daily situations as smoking triggers. These cause you to smoke "just like that," with no reason at all. These situations can create enormous pressure to have a cigarette. As these behavior patterns are stored in the same site of the brain as survival behaviors, this craving can become absurdly strong. But cigarettes are not necessary for your survival.

Also, think of the mice that physically were long since free of nicotine addiction and yet, as an immediate reflex reaction to a light signal, they pressed the lever to get nicotine. This conditioned light signal had to be overcome and separated from nicotine withdrawal. For you, this means the following: In the coming weeks, it could be helpful to somewhat distance yourself from yourself. Look at your own behavior as if you were observing it through a camera filming you from above. You will have to reprogram your mind several times during this period to get rid of everything that triggers you to smoke. As you encounter each trigger, you alone can decide whether you want to continue to smoke or you want to quit. After a few weeks of refusing to give in to them, the triggers will really be gone.

An example: Using the telephone and smoking have nothing to do with each other. This has only been conditioned in your head through the effect of the drug: "Smoke a cigarette; it relaxes me when I'm on the phone and is much more comfortable." Don't fall into that trap again. Remind yourself that cigarettes don´t relax you; on the contrary, they cause additional stress and in 30 minutes you will need another one. Devise a logical counterargument to each excuse you may try to use to give yourself permission to reach for a cigarette. Look at the conversations on pages 141–42 again.

The Lapse Triangle—Never Juggle with More Than One Trigger at a Time

Never try to juggle too many triggers at once. The strongest triggers are other smokers, trouble, and alcohol. Avoid confronting more than one of these triggers in one situation.

"Yeah, another rule from a self–help book. And how did they discover that you should be careful in these trigger situations?" Smokers put all lapses and tempting situations into their smart phones. In this way you can evaluate thousands of these temptation situations and not falsely reconstructed by memory but exactly at the moment when such a situation happened in real life. I repeat. The 3 really significant situations are *other smokers, trouble, and alcohol*.[151] [152] [153] Let all alarm bells ring when these triggers are activated. Often a smoker who is willing to quit can cope with one of these triggers.

Alcohol doubles the risk of having a cigarette lapse in the first weeks. This was shown by the lapses recorded on the smokers' phones.[154] It has also been determined in this manner that trouble or negative stress, which really burdens you, makes you frustrated or places you under pressure, or makes you furious, also leads twice as often to lapses or even relapses.

2 triggers at the same time are very risky. Being around other smokers plus alcohol lowers the level of self-control, and before you know it you have a cigarette in your hand. It's as simple as that. Other smokers plus trouble is another license to lapse. You want immediate relief from negative feelings, and on top of that have smoke from other smokers in your nose as the possible "solution" to your problems.

The killer combination is all 3: Trouble plus other smokers plus alcohol—forget it! If you encounter one of these triggers, avoid it in any circumstance where a second trigger is also present. The lapse triangle is easy to recognize and can be avoided successfully in the first weeks.

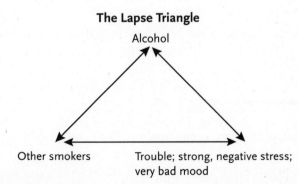

The Lapse Triangle

Alcohol

Other smokers

Trouble; strong, negative stress; very bad mood

Set Clear Rules for Smokers

Does your partner smoke? Then he or she should smoke on the balcony from now on. In the first weeks after quitting, try to avoid smokers or go with them to places where smoking is prohibited. You need friends and distraction during the initial weeks, but make it very clear that they should not smoke in your presence and that they should not offer you a cigarette. Other smokers will respect such clear rules. Above all, they will envy you for the decision you have made because 70% of smokers would like to quit.[155] If you are among smokers, such as at a party, then observe other smokers not with envy but with pity. They have to continue to smoke, because they are hooked. In contrast, you have dared to take the step toward freedom. But in such a situation, under no circumstances should you drink alcohol. Not during the first weeks, until the conditioned urge to smoke when drinking has disappeared.

Avoid Trouble Plus . . .

If you are one of those smokers who smoke particularly in situations where there is trouble, mood swings, or severe stress, you must be extremely careful in these situations. You will often have to develop new strategies to solve problems and to cool off emotionally without following your habit of "smoking away" the situation. You have to find trust in coping with these situations without a cigarette. If you really are confronted with stress and trouble, then avoid the presence of other smokers. Even an otherwise helpful friend smoking away in front of you, when you are in trouble, is a direct incentive to smoke. Makes sense, doesn't it? Remember, never try to juggle 2 of these core triggers at once.

Avoid Alcohol Plus . . .

Avoid alcohol in the first weeks of quitting. This is often coupled with social situations where people smoke. Do not drink alcohol in bars or at parties where smoking is permitted. If you are a social smoker, then you are heavily conditioned to these situations.

Please note that we are concerned here *only* with the initial weeks after quitting. Once you have internalized identifying its 3 factors, the lapse triangle is easy to detect and can be handled really well with sound common sense. It will also show you that consistent situation management has an enormous effect on whether you have a lapse or successfully sidestep the most common triggers.

The Coffee-Cigarette Connection

"I almost reached for a cigarette this morning with my coffee." Coffee is one of the best-conditioned triggers. If you have paired coffee with a cigarette 3 times a day, you have conditioned this situation 11,000 times in a period of 10 years. It is absolutely normal that this conditioning will not leave immediately. Coffee plus nicotine usually gave you energy and brought your mood swings back temporarily to a normal level—until you got the next downer. The risk of falling prey to a coffee-related cigarette lapse increases by over 36% after quitting smoking.[156] So, should you stop drinking coffee? No. Particularly in the first days after quitting, it is more difficult to find your normal drive. During that period, smokers without caffeine are more often exhausted and feel they have no drive. This was tested on 162 coffee-drinking smokers who quit.[157] Caffeine keeps you awake, concentrated, and stimulates. With caffeine, your mood improves. Without caffeine, you also think, "Have a cigarette; at least that will wake you up." My advice for the first days: Change from the conditioned coffee to tea, which also contains caffeine. Even better would be a coffee protein shake. Or try coffee with cold milk or some other form of protein, rather than by itself. In this way you will get your caffeine, but also additional stimulating protein components that quickly build up the metabolism and the production of the happiness transmitters in your body. The metabolism is stimulated by such an extent by protein that some people even perspire slightly after 30 minutes. One thing that is also really great: Your concentration will improve, as protein contains the components for neurotransmitters that stimulate concentration. Coffee shakes and coffee with milk are very rarely conditioned by cigarettes, as cigarettes taste really vile after drinking milk.

ADVICE: Use whey protein in your shakes. In contrast to milk protein, it is more soluble in a shake and reaches the bloodstream faster. Also whey protein, as compared to milk or soy protein, has the highest content of the amino acid tryptophan. This amino acid is the building block for serotonin, one of the main mood-enhancing neurotransmitters. (Read more about protein in chapter 21.)

How Long Does the Craving for Cigarettes Last?

"Forever . . . it feels like hours." Above all, you think initially, "This is always the way it is going to be . . ." But what are the true facts? When craving and its duration was reported by thousands of ex-smokers via their cell phones, the average duration was only 8 minutes. You must bridge this manageable short period. The cravings get less and less. They are like a wave: Either you get washed away or you dive through this wave by using clear logic and your precise aim.

The 3-D Rule

*D*isappear, *D*istract yourself, *D*on´t be impatient:

Those are the best strategies to cope with craving.

DISAPPEAR: Leave the place where you feel the temptation to smoke and go outside. Just a few steps in the fresh air—moving body and spirit—help. Even just opening a window and breathing fresh air as you gaze outside can be a remove.

DISTRACT YOURSELF: Meet friends; talk to someone on the telephone, someone who will support you. Do something—sports, cook, go to the cinema, drink water or tea. Decide to do something in the following days that you wanted to do for a long time and start planning it. Distraction is quite important in the first days and weeks.

> You should always have a portable mini cigarette-butt museum with you (see page 188). Take a sniff. That will usually put an end to your desire for a cigarette.

DON T BE IMPATIENT: Always keep in mind: Such craving attacks usually pass within a short time. The faster you occupy yourself with something else, the faster you will forget the craving.

What to Do When You Have a Lapse

"I smoked a cigarette. I feel that I have failed. I probably won't manage to quit anyway." So, you lit up a cigarette? Okay! It happens. But this does not mean you are now a smoker again. What has happened? You have fallen off the bicycle on a bumpy part in the learning phase. You are in good company: Some 70% of smokers who quit have lapses. Having a lapse is not the same thing as going back to smoking. Get on the bicycle again as quickly as possible:

- Put out the cigarette as soon as you can.
- Make a brief analysis of the situation. What caused

you to smoke? Did you have a really frustrating situation? Did you expect too much of yourself during the first week or 2? Did you have a quarrel with someone who showed no consideration for you? Were others smoking where you were present? Was it a combination of the lapse triangle? Or was it a "just like that" situation where you simply didn't think about what you were doing?

- Do not indulge in self-reproach or "Why will I never manage to quit?" thoughts.
- Reflect quickly on your goals and how much you will benefit from quitting smoking. What should your life look like in 2 to 3 months?
- Think of all the reasons that you no longer want to smoke.
- Look at your list of what you hate about smoking (see page 181).
- Remind yourself of the progress you have made and that you have mastered much more difficult situations in your life. What comes to mind?
- What advice would you give a good friend if he or she was in your situation now?
- Make the decision to recognize and avoid the lapse triangle.
- Think of something that would do you good at this moment instead of smoking.
- Speak to people whom you enjoy.
- Try to reduce stress and give yourself a little break. You do not have to function at 100% in the first 2 weeks. But once you have finally kicked nicotine, you will perform much better.
- Think of yourself frequently in the coming days and simply say no to others' demands. You would do the same if you were recovering from a bad cold.

- You will discover other personal strategies with which you can train in the 30-day Internet program.
- Get up and move on.

Remember: Lapses have nothing to do with failure. They happen. Just in the same way as a top football team has to concede a goal because someone didn't pay attention for a second—that does not mean they've lost the game. Perhaps it was just luck. It happens. Think again about winning. Success feeds on success. This has actually been documented: More than 11,000 kinds of such tempting situations have been evaluated and compared with the subsequent rate of relapse, of going back to smoking. The result: The number of goals you score (the tempting situations avoided) will make you stronger and reduce the risk of future relapse.[158] So every goal counts. Every situation where you did not succumb to temptation is a training unit to decondition your brain. So stop complaining, "Another craving that I cannot bear." Train yourself to think instead, "Aha, a craving. *I'll* show you who's boss." The important thing is that the longer you do not smoke, the less often these defense situations occur. The path in front of you will become smoother and things will take care of themselves. You can succeed. Just in the same way that 8 out of 10 smokers become ex-smokers.

Move On Quickly After a Lapse

So, you smoke a few cigarettes, are disappointed by yourself, and think. "So, now what—I might as well smoke a whole pack." Even in a really bad lapse where you smoke several packs, you should get into the game again. Just because you dropped the ball doesn't mean the goal line has been moved. Keep your eye on the goal.

"I don't even need to try again. I won´t succeed anyway." Do not let such negative feelings bring you down. You've already scored your first victories. You now know the opponent and its tricks. Most smokers have to make several attempts at quitting. They fall on their face a few times and still succeed in the end. You do not want to inhale toxic substances for the rest of your life. Smoking is of no benefit to your well-being. It helps to recall this to mind time and time again. You cannot read chapters 8 to 10 often enough!

Make Another Attempt

"I am sure I am one of those smokers who has had a complete relapse!" Stop. That is exactly what your addicted brain wants you to believe. But what is the difference between smokers who have a relapse and those who don't? Weakness? No. Think of the thousands of slips, lapses, and relapses that were reported by smokers via their smart phones and were compared. The most noticeable thing was: Smokers who did not have a relapse were usually just lucky in not being confronted with tempting situations or by managing to avoid them. That sounds amazing at first. But in the first weeks, the trick is to avoid juggling too many balls at the same time. Not having contact with other smokers, stress, or alcohol. You should consciously manage this lapse triangle. The rest you can handle with the right antilapse strategies. Perhaps you should try nicotine patches or other medication, if the lapse took place during the first 2 weeks of physical withdrawal. Open yourself to accepting a little help. In fact many who have managed to quit said, "It wasn't easy, but a lot easier than I thought." Everyone can make it. All dictators are eventually tumbled from power.

THE 30-DAY PROGRAM

These have been just a few pieces of advice to manage lapses and craving situations. Using the learning program, you can train yourself to continue and also to motivate yourself: Look at the documentation on smoking, download relaxation exercises, and meet other smokers in the forum. In this way, you remain close to your personal goals and the reasons why you want to quit and how you can cope with craving situations.

Nonsmokers: Never Try Another Cigarette

You've managed to become a nonsmoker. Stay that way! Some ex-smokers try a cigarette after 6 months because they are certain that *this* one cigarette won't matter. That's difficult because . . . there is no such thing as *one* cigarette. You can never become *just* a social smoker—kiss that fantasy good-bye.

You have memories that for many years have been firmly coupled with memories of smoking. That is okay. It is a part of your life. At the beginning, during the first year after quitting, you may experience a short nostalgia for smoking. But look at this memory for what it is: Nostalgia for smoking does not feel like a craving. It is more like a fleeting thought that passes just as quickly. Please never fall into the nostalgia trap. ("Ah, a cigarette can do no harm . . . then I'll stop again. I am a nonsmoker and I don't miss it.") There is no such thing as just one cigarette! Even a small amount of nicotine will set off the chain reaction again: As soon as the nicotine wears off, a little voice will whisper in your ear, "Smoke another one." If you fall for this, the nicotine trap will snap shut mercilessly, imprisoning you once again in your old addiction.

The classic story is: You have become a nonsmoker but, "just

290

for the sake of it," have smoked one with friends. Is that a relapse? No. It is stupidity and has nothing to do with a relapse. And every smoker has told me the exact same story. "Then, unfortunately, I tried one. Disgusting . . . it was easy to stop . . . and then somehow I felt like another one . . . and now I am smoking again." This single cigarette costs you thousands of dollars as soon as you set off this chain reaction again. It is important to know that nostalgia for cigarettes wears off the longer you are a non-smoker. It is nothing more than a fleeting thought. But if you take a nicotine fix, this means more years of slavery to cigarettes.

> **The most important rule at the end of this book: Once you've stopped smoking, please never try even one single cigarette again!**

THE BOTTOM LINE

- ▸ Drugs condition normal situations into smoking triggers. It takes some weeks to get rid of these.
- ▸ At the beginning be careful not to juggle the following 3 triggers all at once: others who smoke + alcohol + trouble/stress.
- ▸ Use the 3-D Rule: Disappear, Distract yourself, Don´t be impatient.
- ▸ Lapses are neither a failure nor a relapse. Accept this. Stub out the cigarette and continue on the path to become a nonsmoker.
- ▸ When you are a nonsmoker, never try a single cigarette again.

30

Your Personal Care and Support

IN EVERY COUNTRY, VARIOUS TELEPHONE hotlines that offer excellent advice and help in every situation are usually sponsored by the state. Learn more about free services available in your area.

"I'M STILL NOT 100% SURE . . . I WOULD PREFER TO SPEAK TO SOMEONE." Before their last cigarette, many have personal questions. On the smoker hotlines, you can discuss everything personally, to feel more secure. Those who staff such lines understand that every smoker is different.

"AH, I DON'T FEEL COMFORTABLE WITH THAT." Why not? You are anonymous and you can say whatever you want. The advisers are true professionals, and provide confidentiality. That's what makes their advice different from the good advice of friends.

"I AM SURE I WOULD HAVE TO KEEP MYSELF SHORT." Usually hotlines have no time limit, as they are sponsored by the state. The conversation can last 20 to 30 minutes, until all your doubts have been taken care of.

"YEAH, THAT'S ONE THING, SPEAKING WITH A GOOD COUNSELOR. THEN THE NEXT TIME, THERE IS SOMEONE ELSE ON THE OTHER END AND I HAVE TO START AGAIN FROM THE BEGINNING." Do you want a personal contact person who perhaps listens frequently to what you have to say and to hear how things are going? Without you having to call again yourself? It is precisely for this reason that many countries offer hotlines via which you can arrange automatic callbacks. Your questions immediately before quitting will be very different than those during the first week after you have quit, when you may want to know how to cope with withdrawal symptoms, or after 3 weeks, when you may simply need some moral support to keep going. Checking in with the same person who truly cares about your progress is exciting.

"DOES THAT REALLY HELP? A FEW CONVERSATIONS?" A good question. Of course, there have been assessments of how effective telephone hotlines are: Over 24,000 individual consultations and 9 studies have been evaluated.[159][160] The result: With the telephone support, more smokers manage to quit. Several calls from someone who is personally supporting you are better than just one call.

"CAN I ALSO CALL WHEN I AM JUST ABOUT TO SMOKE A CIGARETTE?" Certainly, please do. Even a short conversation can make you think differently. That is why the hotline counselors are there. It is best to store their emergency numbers in your phone's directory, for just such a situation.

"I DO NOT KNOW IF I CAN CONTINUALLY BOTHER THE COUNSELOR." Yes, you can. And you do not need to have a bad conscience. For in spite of tobacco tax and the savings in pensions, smokers cost your government more than it earns from your smoking. A hotline is not a charity; it pays off for the state. So make full use of this offer. That is why the hotlines are there.

"I ALREADY HAVE CANCER FROM SMOKING. IS IT WORTH STOPPING NOW?" Yes, it is always worth it. The function of the immune system will greatly improve as will general wellbeing. Many countries have a special hotline for smokers with cancer. Enter into a search engine: "Cancer smoking hotline."

Seminars

So, you need more direct contact and motivation? Then a seminar could be the answer for you. Group seminars double your chances of quitting.[161] The direct exchange with the trainer and other smokers wishing to quit provides enormous motivation. You see how all smokers face the same problems as you do and on this day you will smoke your last cigarette.

Studies show that online seminars can also double your chance of quitting! The online program "My 30 day quit smoking coach" has been carefully designed by experienced non-smoking coaches to meet all the aspects that you may encounter when you quit. An upgrade to the premium version of the online seminar gives you a full 30 days of support and you can meet other smokers in the chat room to exchange ideas and support one another.

THE BOTTOM LINE

- ▶ Personal help and support from government-sponsored hotlines provides you with additional help.
- ▶ You can make use of these hotlines exactly when you need them, whether you are just about to lapse or need to receive prearranged phone calls from your own personal counselor.
- ▶ Quitting seminars are effective. The personal exchange with the trainer and the group provide enormous motivation.

Login and Password
for the Online Program

As a reader you can login for free for the first 10 days of the online program.

These are the ten units of the program *before* you quit.

 Register at: www.my30dayquitsmokingcoach.com
Login name: smokefree
Password: freedom

A Final Word

- **NEVER DOUBT YOUR DECISION TO QUIT SMOKING!**
- **REMIND YOURSELF CONSTANTLY THAT NICOTINE HAS NOT A SINGLE BENEFIT FOR YOUR MIND.**
  It does not reduce stress nor does it improve your mood. Nicotine causes stress, mood swings, and problems in concentration by changing the reward system in the brain. It makes you unstable and susceptible to these negative feelings.
- **ALWAYS KEEP IN MIND THAT YOU ONLY "LIKE" SMOKING TO AVOID AND RELIEVE THE NERVOUS FEELING OF EMPTINESS AND THE RESTLESSNESS OF WITHDRAWAL.**
  Nicotine has not a single benefit for your well-being except in that it relieves your withdrawal symptoms. Quit and this one final withdrawal that you may experience now for 2 to 3 weeks will be your last craving period. Otherwise nicotine will pressure you little by little every day. For the rest of your life! And you will experience that withdrawal more frequently as the places where smoking is permitted are becoming fewer and fewer.
- **BELIEVE ME: YOU WILL SOON FEEL MUCH MORE STABLE WITHOUT NICOTINE.**
  In a few weeks you will no longer crave a cigarette. You will feel less stressed, more awake, and full of energy in the morning. You will be able to concentrate for longer periods of time, have a more stable mood,

and feel physically fitter. You have escaped from the lethal smoking torture chamber.

- **TAKE PLEASURE IN YOUR NEWFOUND FREEDOM.**
  You are not giving up anything. On the contrary: You are regaining your freedom. You will be proud of yourself. Welcome to a life beyond the bonds of addiction. Look forward to it.

- **WHEN YOU HAVE BECOME A NONSMOKER, NEVER TRY A SINGLE CIGARETTE AGAIN.**

- **HELPING OTHERS QUIT ALSO HELPS YOU.**
  If this book has helped you, please recommend it to other smokers. This may help them quit smoking. Helping others quit also helps you never to smoke again. As well as this, you are also damaging the nicotine dealers who have taken so much money from you for such a long time. This big business with death only works as long as you continue to smoke.

Yours,
Andreas Jopp

Endnotes

1   L. Shahab and R. West, "Do Ex-Smokers Report Feeling Happier Following Cessation? Evidence from a Cross-sectional Survey," *Nicotine & Tobacco Research* 11, no. 5 (2009): 553–57.

2   Y. A. Abreu-Villaca et al., "Short Term Adolescent Nicotine Exposure Has Immediate and Persistent Effects on Cholinergic Systems: Critical Periods, Patterns of Exposure, Dose Thresholds," *Neuropsychopharmacology* 28 (2003): 1935–49.

3   E. T. Moolchan, M. Ernst, and J. E. Henningfield, "A Review of Tobacco Smoking in Adolescents: Treatment Implications," *Journal of the American Academy of Child and Adolescent Psychiatry* 39 (2000): 682–93.

4   Selected documents from the Legacy Tobacco Documents Library, http://legacy.library.ucsf.edu/tid/eyn18c00.

5   Selected documents from the Legacy Tobacco Documents Library, http://legacy.library.ucsf.edu/tid/lve76b00

6   K.-O. Haustein and D. Groneberg, *Tabakabhängigkeit* (Berlin: Springer 2008), 620–21.

7   Molly Human. Female Celebrity Smoking List, at Smoking sides. com, http://smokingsides.com/asfs/m/most.html.

8   J. Sargent et al., "Brand Appearances in Contemporary Cinema Films and Contribution to Global Marketing of Cigarettes," *The Lancet* 357 (2001): 29–32.

9   C. Mekemson and S. Grant, "How the Tobacco Industry Built Its Relationship with Hollywood," *Tobacco Control* 11 (2002): i181–i191.

10 R. Hanewinkel and J. D. Sargent, "Exposure to Smoking in Internationally Distributed American Movies and Youth Smoking in Germany: A Cross-cultural Cohort Study," *Pediatrics* 121 (2008): 108–17.

11 M. A. Dalton et al., "Effect of Viewing Smoking in Movies on Adolescent Smoking Initiation: A Cohort Study," *The Lancet* 362 (2009): 281–85.

12 B. S. Fagg et al., "Rest Program Review," RJReynolds Company, May 3, 1991, Legacy Library, http://legacy.library.ucsf.edu/tid/gpi73d00.

13 K. O. Haustein and D. Groneberg, *Tabakabhängigkeit* (Berlin: Springer 2008), 56–57.

14 G. N. Connolly et al., "Trends in Nicotine Yield in Smoke and Its Relationship with Design Characteristics Among Popular US Cigarette Brands, 1997–2005," *Tobacco Control* 16 (2007): e5.

15   R. Pollay and T. Dewhirst, "The Dark Side of Marketing Seemingly 'Light' Cigarettes: Successful Images and Failed Fact," *Tobacco Control* 11 (2002): 20.

16   H. Tindle et al., "Cessation Among Smokers of 'Light' Cigarettes: Results from the 2000 National Health Interview Survey," *American Journal of Public Health* 96 (2006): 1498–1504.

17   K.-O. Haustein and D. Groneberg, *Tabakabhängigkeit* (Berlin: Springer 2008), 56.

18   M. A. H. Russell et al., "Comparison of Effect on Tobacco Consumption and Carbon Monoxide Absorption of Changing to High and Low Nicotine Cigarettes," *BMJ* 4 (1973): 512–16.

19   Translator's note: This quote is retranslated from the German edition of the book. C. E. Teague, "Research Planning Memorandum on the Nature of Tobacco Business and the Crucial Role of Nicotine Therein," 1972, Bates No. 500915683-5691.

20   R. V. Fant, K. J. Schuh, and M. L. Stitzer, "Response to Smoking as a Function of Prior Smoking Amounts," *Psychopharmacology* 119, no. 4 (1995): 385–90.

21   K. J. Schuh, "Desire to Smoke During Spaced Smoking Intervals," *Psychopharmacology* 120, no. 3 (1995): 289–95.

22   D. S. Burrows, M. L. Orlowsky, and H. J. Lees, "Younger Adult Smokers: Strategies and Opportunities," February 29, 1984, Bates: 501928462-501928550; http://tobaccodocuments.org/rjr/501928462-8550.html.

23   T. S. Roy, F. J. Seidler, and T. A. Slotkin, "Prenatal Nicotine Exposure Evokes Alterations of Cell Structure in Hippocampus and Somatosensory Cortex," *Journal of Pharmacology and Experimental Therapeutics* 300, no. 1 (2002): 124–33.

24   K. M. Linnet et al., "Maternal Lifestyle Factors in Pregnancy Risk of Attention Deficit Hyperactivity Disorder and Associated Behaviors: Review of the Current Evidence," *American Journal of Psychiatry* 160 (2003):1028–40.

25   K. M. Linnet et al., "Smoking During Pregnancy and the Risk for Hyperkinetic Disorder in Offspring," *Pediatrics* 116, no. 2 (2005): 462–67.

26   R. P. Martin et al., "Smoking During Pregnancy: Association with Childhood Temperament, Behavior, and Academic Performance," *Journal of Pediatric Psychology* 31, no. 5 (2006): 490–500.

27   S. M. Milberger, R. M. Davis, and A. L. Holm, "Pet Owners' Attitudes and Behaviors Related to Smoking and Second-hand Smoke: A Pilot Study," *Tobacco Control* 18 (2009): 156–58.

28   "Raucherkinder ähnlich belastet wie einst Barkeeper," *Die Welt*, October 27, 2010.

29   "Wer qualmt schadet sich doppelt," Focus online, January 20, 2010.

30   Deutsches Krebsforschungszentrum, *Tabakatlas Deutschsland 2009* (Heidelberg: Steinkopff, 2009), 48.

31   E. R. Bertone, L. A. Snyder, and A. S. Moore, "Environmental Tobacco Smoke and Risk of Malignant Lymphoma in Pet Cats," *American Journal of Epidemiology* 156 (2002): 268–73.

32   J. S. Reif, C. Bruns, and K. S. Lower, "Cancer of the Nasal Cavity and Paranasal Sinuses and Exposure to Environmental Tobacco Smoke in Pet Dogs," *American Journal of Epidemiology* 147, no. 5 (1998): 488–92.

33   F. F. Ikard, D. E. Green, and D. Horn, "A Scale to Differentiate Between Types of Smoking as Related to the Management of the Affect," *Addiction* 4 (1969): 649–59.

34   A. C. Parrott, "Acute Pharmacodynamic Tolerance to the Subjective Effects of Cigarette Smoking," *Psychopharmacology* 116 (1994): 93–97.

35   J. A. Fidler and R. West, "Self-Perceived Smoking Motives and Their Correlates in a General Population Sample," *Nicotine & Tobacco Research* 11, no. 10 (2009): 1182–88.

36   A. C. Parrott and N. J. Garnham, "Comparative Mood States and Cognitive Skills of Cigarette Smokers, Deprived Smokers and Nonsmokers," *Psychopharmacology* 13, no. 5 (1998): 367–76.

37   A. C. Parrott and F. J. Kaye, "Daily Uplifts, Hassles, Stresses and Cognitive Failures: In Cigarette Smokers, Abstaining Smokers, and Nonsmokers," *Behavioral Pharmacology* 10 (1999): 639–46.

38   K. Aronson et al., "Smoking Is Associated with Worse Mood on Stressful Days: Results from a National Diary Study," *Annals of Behavioral Medicine* 36, no. 3 (2008): 259–69.

39   M. Herbert et al., "No Effect of Cigarette Smoking on Attention or Mood in Nondeprived Smokers," *Addiction* 96 (2001): 1349–56.

40   A. C. Parrott, "Nesbitt's Paradox Resolved? Stress and Arousal Modulation During Cigarette Smoking," *Addiction* 98 (1998): 27–39.

41   A. Adan, G. Prat, and M. Sánchez-Turet, "Effects of Nicotine Dependence on Diurnal Variations of Subjective Activation and Mood," *Addiction* 99, no. 12 (2004): 1599–1607.

42   A. C. Parrott, "Cigarette Smoking and Abstinence: Comparative Effects upon Cognitive Task Performance and Mood State over 24 Hours," *Human Psychopharmacology* 11 (1996): 391–400.

43   M. Herbert, J. Foulds, and C. Fife-Schaw, "No Effect of Cigarette Smoking on Attention or Mood in Non-deprived Smokers," *Addiction* 96 (2001): 1349–56.

44   A. Parrott et al., "Comparative Mood States and Cognitive Skills of Cigarette Smokers, Deprived Smokers and Non-smokers," *Psychopharmacology* 13, no. 5 (1998): 367–76.

45   K. Soar et al., "The Effects of Cigarette Smoking and Abstinence on Auditory Verbal Learning," *Human Psychopharmacology* 23 (2008): 621–27.

46   R. Scragg et al., "Diminished Autonomy over Tobacco Can Appear with the First Cigarettes," *Addictive Behaviors* 33 (2008): 689–98.

47   Y. A. Abreu-Villaça et al., "Short Term Adolescent Nicotine Exposure Has

Immediate and Persistent Effects on Cholinergic Systems: Critical Periods, Patterns of Exposure, Dose Thresholds," *Neuropsychopharmacology* 28 (2003): 1935–49.

48   J. R. DiFranza et al., "Symptoms of Tobacco Dependence After Brief Intermittent Use," *Archives of Pediatric & Adolescent Medicine* 161, no. 7 (2007): 704–10.

49   M. O. Chaiton et al., "A Systematic Review of Longitudinal Studies on the Association Between Depression and Smoking in Adolescents," *BMC Public Health* 9 (2009): 356.

50   Ibid.

51   G. C. Patton et al., "Depression, Anxiety, and Smoking Initiation: A Prospective Study over 3 Years," *American Journal of Public Health* 88, no. 10 (1998): 1518–22.

52   A. C. Parrott, "Cigarette-Derived Nicotine Is Not a Medicine," *World Journal of Biological Psychiatry* 4 (2003): 49–55.

53   J. R. Hughes, "Tobacco Withdrawal in Self-Quitters," *Journal of Consulting and Clinical Psychology* 60 (1992): 689–97.

54   M. P. Carey et al., "Stress and Unaided Smoking Cessation: A Prospective Investigation," *Journal of Consulting and Clinical Psychology* 61 (1993): 831–38.

55   S. Cohen and E. Lichtenstein, "Perceived Stress, Quitting Smoking, and Smoking Relapse," *Health Psychology* 9 (1990): 466–78.

56   R. West and P. Hajek, "What Happens to Anxiety Levels on Giving Up Smoking?" *American Journal of Psychiatry* 154 (1997): 1589–92.

57   I. Lang et al., "Was John Reid Right? Smoking, Class, and Pleasure: A Population-Based Cohort Study in England," *Public Health* 121, no. 7 (2007): 518–24.

58   L. Shahab and R. West, "Do Ex-Smokers Report Feeling Happier Following Cessation? Evidence from a Cross-sectional Survey," *Nicotine & Tobacco Research* 11, no. 5 (2009): 553–57.

59   A. C. Parrott, "Acute Pharmacodynamic Tolerance to the Subjective Effects of Cigarette Smoking," *Psychopharmacology* 116 (1994): 93–97.

60   A. C. Parrott and N. J. Garnham, "Comparative Mood States and Cognitive Skills of Cigarette Smokers, Deprived Smokers and Nonsmokers," *Psychopharmacology* 13, no. 5 (1998): 367–76.

61   A. C. Parrott and F. J. Kaye, "Daily Uplifts, Hassles, Stresses and Cognitive Failures: In Cigarette Smokers, Abstaining Smokers, and Nonsmokers," *Behavioral Pharmacology* 10 (1999): 639–46.

62   S. Cohen and E. Lichtenstein, "Perceived Stress, Quitting Smoking, and Smoking Relapse," *Health Psychology* 9 (1990): 466–78.

63   D. J. K. Balfour, "The Neurobiology of Tobacco Dependence: A Preclinical Perspective on the Role of the Dopamine Projections to the Nucleus," *Nicotine & Tobacco Research* 6, no. 6 (2004): 899–912.

64   M. G. LeSage et al., "Reinstatement of Nicotine Self-Administration

in Rats by Presentation of Nicotine-Paired Stimuli, but Not Nicotine Priming," *Pharmacology Biochemistry and Behavior* 79 (2004): 507–13.

65   R. F. Mucha et al., "Modulation of Craving by Cues Having Differential Overlap with Pharmacological Effect: Evidence for Cue Approach in Smokers and Social Drinkers," *Psychopharmacology* 147 (1999): 306–13.

66   A. R. Caggiula et al., "Cue Dependency of Nicotine Self-Administration and Smoking," *Pharmacology Biochemistry and Behavior* 70 (2001): 515–30.

67   A. R. Caggiula et al., "Environmental Stimuli Promote the Acquisition of Nicotine Self-Administration in Rats," *Psychopharmacology* (Berlin) 163 (2002): 230–37.

68   N. E. Paterson, W. Froestl, and A. Markou, "Repeated Administration of the GABAB Receptor Agonist CGP44532 Decreased Nicotine Self-Administration, and Acute Administration Decreased Cue-Induced Reinstatement of Nicotine-Seeking in Rats," *Neuropsychopharmacology* 30 (2005): 119–28.

69   C. Cohen et al., "Nicotine-Associated Cues Maintain Nicotine-Seeking Behavior in Rats Several Weeks After Nicotine Withdrawal: Reversal by the Cannabinoid (CB1) Receptor Antagonist, Rimonabant (SR141716)," *Neuropsychopharmacology* 30 (2005): 145–55.

70   X. Liu et al., "Reinstatement of Nicotine-Seeking Behavior by Drug-Associated Stimuli After Extinction in Rats," *Psychopharmacology* (Berlin) 184, no. 3–4 (March 2006): 417–25.

71   K. A. O'Connell, J. E. Schwartz, and S. Shiffman, "Do Resisted Temptations During Smoking Cessation Deplete or Augment Self-Control Resources?," *Psychology of Addictive Behaviors* 22, no. 4 (2008): 486–95.

72   K.-O. Haustein and D. Groneberg, *Tabakabhängigkeit* (Berlin: Springer 2008), 565.

73   T. Duesing, "Machen Zigaretten unsympathisch," *Men's Health*, April 20, 2006.

74   Wikipedia, "Tabakrauch," December 7, 2010.

75   Deutsches Krebsforschungszentrum, *Tabakatlas Deutschland 2009*, 18.

76   R. Chari et al., "Effect of Active Smoking on the Human Bronchial Epithelium Transcriptome," *BMC Genomics* 8 (2007): 297.

77   List of cigarette carcinogens, http://en.wikipedia.org/wiki/Smoke_constituents.

78   K.-O. Haustein and D. Groneberg, *Tabakabhängigkeit* (Berlin: Springer 2008), 382–85.

79   Ibid., 376–82.

80   M. Risch, "Rauch wie 250 Röntgenaufnahmen pro Jahr," *Süddeutsche Zeitung* (Munich), May 25, 2004.

81   Grenzwerte der World Nuclear Association, http://world-nuclear.org/info/default.aspx?id=486&terms=mSv%2fyr.

82   "Konzerne erhöhen die Nikotindosis in Zigaretten," *Spiegel* magazine, January 18, 2007; cited study: G. N. Connolly et al., "How Cigarette Additives Are Used to Mask Environmental Tobacco Smoke," *Tobacco Control* 9 (2000): 283–91.

83   K. Röske et al., "Prävalenz des Rauchens vor und während der Schwangerschaft—populationsbasierte Daten / Prevalence of Smoking in Women Before and During Pregnancy: Population-Based Data, *"Deutsche Medizinische Wochenschrift* 133, no. 15 (2008):764–68.

84   Deutsche Hauptstelle für Suchtfragen, *Tabakabhängigkeit*, vol. 2 (Hamm: Deutsche Hauptstelle für Suchtfragen, 2003), 24.

85   Marianne Tritz, "Cheflobbyistin des Deutschen Zigarettenverbandes (DZV)," N24-TV talk show *Zu Gast bei Friedmann*, July 8, 2010.

86   R. Doll et al., "Mortality in Relation to Smoking: 50 Years' Observations on Male British Doctors," *BMJ* 328, no. 7455 (2004): 1519.

87   Deutsches Krebsforschungszentrum, *Tabakatlas Deutschland 2009*, 41.

88   Deutsche Hauptstelle für Suchtfragen, *Tabakabhängigkeit*, 27.

89   Haustein and Groneberg, *Tabakabhängigkeit*, 330.

90   E. Radzikowska, P. Głaz, and K. Roszkowski. "Lung Cancer in Women: Age, Smoking, Histology, Performance Status, Stage, Initial Treatment and Survival," *Annals of Oncology* 13, no. 7 (2002): 1087–93.

91   H. Brønnum-Hansen and K. Juel, "Health Life Years Lost Due to Smoking," *Ugeskr Laeger* 164 (2002): 3953–58.

92   P. Boyle, "Cancer, Cigarette Smoking and Premature Death in Europe: A Review Including the Recommendations of European Cancer Experts Consensus Meeting, Helsinki, October 1996," *Lung Cancer* 17 (1997): 1–60.

93   K. A. Perkins et al., "Tobacco Withdrawal in Women and Menstrual Cycle Phase," *Journal of Consulting and Clinical Psychology* 68, no. 1 (2009): 176–80.

94   B. Borelli and M. Mermelstein, "The Role of Weight Concern and Self Efficacy in Smoking Cessation and Weight Gain Among Smokers in a Clinic-Based Cessation Program," *Addictive Behaviors* 23 (1998): 609–22;

95   A. W. Meyers et al., "Are Weight Concerns Predictive of Smoking Cessation? A Prospective Analysis," *Journal of Consulting and Clinical Psychiatry* 65 (1997):448–52.

96   K.-O. Haustein and D. Groneman, *Tabakabhängigkeit*, 2nd ed. (Heidelberg: Springerverlag, 2008), 566–67.

97   Ibid., 563–64.

98   R. C. Klesges et al., "The Prospective Relationship of Smoking and Weight in a Young Biracial Cohort," *Journal of Consulting and Clinical Psychology* 66 (1998): 987–93.

99   F. J. Basterra-Gortari et al., "Effect of Smoking on Body Weight: Longitudinal Analysis of the SUN Cohort," *Revista Española de Cardiología* 63, no. 1 (2010): 20–27.

100 D. Canoy et al., "Cigarette Smoking and Fat Distribution in 21,828 British Men and Women: A Population-Based Study," *Obesity Research* 13, no. 8 (2005): 1466–75.

101 W. Scherbaum et al., "Rauchen und Passivrauchen verursachen Typ 2 Diabetes," *Deutsches Krebsforschungszentrum*, 2008, http://www.dkfz.de/de/tabakkontrolle/download/Publikationen/FzR/FzR_Diabetes.pdf.

102 K. O. Haustein and D. Groneman, *Tabakabhängigkeit*, 2nd ed. (Heidelberg: Springerverlag, 2008), 565.

103 C. S. Pomerleau and K. Saules, "Body Image, Body Satisfaction, and Eating Patterns in Normal-Weight and Overweight/Obese Women Current Smokers and Never-Smokers," *Addictive Behaviors* 32 (2007): 2329–34.

104 C. S. Pomerleau, A. N. Zucker, and A. J. Stewart, "Characterizing Concerns About Post-Cessation Weight Gain: Results from a National Survey of Women Smokers," *Nicotine & Tobacco Research* 3, no. 1 (2001): 51–60.

105 Deutsches Krebsforschungzentrum, "Rauchfrei ohne Gewichtsprobleme," April 7, 2010, www.dkfz.de/de/rauchertelefon/Gewichts probleme.html.

106 B. G. Hoebel et al., "Natural Addiction: A Behavioral and Circuit Model Based on Sugar Addiction in Rats," *Journal of Addiction Medicine* 3 (2009): 33–41.

107 R. L. Corwin and P. S. Grigson, "Symposium Overview—Food Addiction: Fact or Fiction?," *Journal of Nutrition* 139 (2009): 617–19.

108 A. Hanjal, G. P. Smith, and R. Norgren, "Oral Sucrose Stimulation Increases Accumbens Dopamine in the Rat," *American Journal of Physiology. Regulatory Integrative and Comparative Physiology.* 286, no. 1 (2004): R31–37.

109 G. J. Wang et al., "Similarity Between Obesity and Drug Addiction as Assessed by Neurofunctional Imaging: A Concept Review," *Journal of Addictive Diseases* 23 (2004): 39–53.

110 C. Colantuoni et al., "Evidence That Intermittent, Excessive Sugar Intake Causes Endogenous Opioid Dependence," *Obesity Research* 10, no. 6 (2002): 478–88.

111 M. Lenoir et al., "Intense Sweetness Surpasses Cocaine Reward," *PLoS ONE* 2, no. 8 (2007): e698.

112 C. Colantuoni et al., "Evidence That Intermittent, Excessive Sugar Intake Causes Endogenous Opioid Dependence," *Obesity Research* 10, no. 6 (2002): 478–88.

113 N. M. Avena, P. Rada, and B. G. Hoebel, "Evidence for Sugar Addiction: Behavioral and Neurochemical Effects of Intermittent, Excessive Sugar Intake," *Neuroscience & Behavioral Reviews* 32, no. 1 (2008): 20–39.

114 Wang, et al., "Similarity Between Obesity and Drug Addiction as Assessed by Neurofunctional Imaging: A Concept Review," 39–53.

115 B. G. Hoebel et al., "Natural Addiction: A Behavioral and Circuit Model Based on Sugar Addiction in Rats," *Journal of Addiction Medicine* 3 (2009): 33–41.

116 M. Lenoir et al., "Intense Sweetness Surpasses Cocaine Reward," *PLoS ONE* 2, no. 8 (2007): e698.

117 I. Tietjen, "Milch und Obst verderben Rauchgenuss," *Men's Health* April 6, 2007.

118 A. Grahl, "Süßstoffe—süß und sicher," *DGE-aktuell*, August 8, 2007.

119 D. Lauderdale et al., "Body Mass Index in a US National Sample of Asian Americans: Effects of Nativity, Years Since Immigration and Socioeconomic Status," *International Journal of Obesity* 24 (2000): 1188–94.

120 C. Schweizer, A. Schlarb, and D. Revenstorf, "Hypnotherapeutische Raucherentwöhnung in Gruppen: Experimentelle und klinische Hypnose," *Sonderdruck* 17, no. 1 (2001): 61–99.

121 Ibid.

122 Ibid.

123 Ibid.

124 Ibid. (Pedersen, 1975).

125 Ibid. (Watkins, 1976).

126 Ibid. (MacHovec, 1978).

127 Ibid. (Stanton, 1978).

128 Ibid. (Javel, 1980).

129 Ibid. (Barbasz, 1984).

130 Ibid. (Williams, 1988).

131 Ibid. (Heumann, 1988).

132 Ibid. (Schulte, 2000).

133 Ibid. (Cardona 2000).

134 Ibid. (Schweizer, 2001).

135 K.-O. Haustein and D. Groneman, *Tabakabhängigkeit*, 2nd ed. (Heidelberg: Springerverlag, 2008), 79.

136 J. R. Hughes et al., "A Meta-Analysis of the Efficacy of Over-the-Counter Nicotine Replacement," *Tobacco Control* 12 (2003): 21–27.

137 R. A. Walsh, "Over-the-Counter Nicotine Replacement Therapy: A Methodological Review of the Evidence Supporting Its Effectiveness," *Drug and Alcohol Review* 27, no. 5 (2008): 529–47.

138 J. F. Etter et al., "The Impact of Pharmaceutical Company Funding on Results of Randomized Trials of Nicotine Replacement Therapy for Smoking Cessation: A Meta-Analysis," *Addiction* 102, no. 5 (2007): 815–22.

139 B. Shamasunder and L. Bero, "Financial Ties and Conflicts of Interest Between Pharmaceutical and Tobacco Companies," *JAMA* 288 (2002): 738–44.

140 S. Chapmann S. and R. MacKenzie, "The Global Research Neglect of Unassisted Smoking Cessation: Causes and Consequences," *PLoS Medicine* 7, no. 2 (2010): e1000216.

141 L. F. Stead et al., "Nicotine Replacement Therapy for Smoking Cessation," *Cochrane Database of Systematic Reviews* 3 (2008): 1.

142 Adapted from K.-O. Haustein and D. Groneman, *Tabakabhängigkeit*, 2nd ed. (Heidelberg: Springerverlag, 2008), 520–21. Note: Nicotine nasal spray has been taken off the market in many countries on account of its addiction potential. Therefore it has not been included in the table.

143 P. Puska et al., "Combined Use of Nicotine Patch and Gum Compared with Gum Alone in Smoking Cessation: A Clinical Trial in North Karelia," *Tobacco Control* 4, no. 3 (1995): 231–35.

144 Deutsche Hauptstelle für Suchtfragen, *Tabakabhängigkeit*, vol. 2: 81.

145 A. R. White et al., "Acupuncture and Related Interventions for Smoking Cessation," *Cochrane Database of Systematic Reviews* 25, no. 1 (2006).

146 D. Gonzales et al., "Varenicline, an alpha4beta2 Nicotinic Acetylcholine Receptor Partial Agonist, vs Sustained-Release Bupropion and Placebo for Smoking Cessation: A Randomized Controlled Trial," *JAMA* 296 (2006): 47–55.

147 H. J. Aubin et al., "Varenicline Versus Transdermal Nicotine Patch for Smoking Cessation: Results from a Randomised Open-Label Trial," *Thorax* 63, no. 8 (2008): 717–24.

148 Gonzales et al., "Varenicline, an alpha4beta2 Nicotinic Acetylcholine Receptor Partial Agonist, vs Sustained-Release Bupropion and Placebo for Smoking Cessation: A Randomized Controlled Trial," 47–55.

149 K. Fagerström et al., "Varenicline in the Treatment of Tobacco Dependence," *Neuropsychiatric Disease Treatment* 4, no. 2 (2008): 353–63.

150 "FDA Warnung zum Raucherentwöhnungsmittel Champix," *Deutsches Ärzteblatt*, February 5, 2008, www.aerzteblatt.de/v4/news/news.asp?id=31284.

151 S. Shiffman et al., "First Lapses to Smoking: Within-Subjects Analysis of Real-Time Reports," *Journal of Consulting and Clinical Psychology* 64, no. 2 (1996): 366–79. Note: Small portable computers were used. I described them as smart phones in this consumer book.

152 S. Shiffman et al., "Temptations to Smoke After Quitting: A Comparison of Lapsers and Maintainers," *Health Psychology* 15, no. 6 (1996): 455–61.

153 S. Shiffman et al., "Prediction of Lapse from Associations Between Smoking and Situational Antecedents Assessed by Ecological Momentary Assessment," *Drug and Alcohol Dependency* 91, no. 2–3 (2007): 159–68.

154 Ibid.

155 Centers for Disease Control and Prevention (CDC), "Cigarette Smoking Among Adults—United States, 2000," *Morbidity & Mortality Weekly Report* 51 (2002): 642–45.

156   S. Shiffman et al., "Prediction of Lapse from Associations Between Smoking and Situational Antecedents Assessed by Ecological Momentary Assessment," *Drug and Alcohol Dependency* 91, no. 2–3 (2007): 159–68.

157   J. A. Swanson et al., "The Impact of Caffeine Use on Tobacco Cessation and Withdrawal," *Addictive Behaviors* 22 (1997): 55–68.

158   K. A. O'Connell, J. E. Schwartz, and S. Shiffman, "Do Resisted Temptations During Smoking Cessation Deplete or Augment Self-Control Resources?," *Psychology of Addictive Behaviors* 22, no. 4 (2008): 486–95.

159   L. F. Stead, R. Perera, and T. Lancaster, "Telephone Counseling for Smoking Cessation," *Cochrane Database of Systematic Reviews* 3 2009, art. no. CD002850.

160   L. F. Stead et al., "A Systematic Review of Interventions for Smokers Who Contact Quitlines," *Tobacco Control* 16 (2007): 3–8.

161   L. F. Stead and T. Lancaster, "Group Behaviour Therapy Programmes for Smoking Cessation," *Cochrane Database of Systematic Reviews* 2 (2005).

PUBLISHER'S NOTE:

In adapting *I Know You Like to Smoke but You Can Quit—Now* the publisher independently elected to reformat the endnotes in a style that is used widely in American publishing but that diverges from the German original, which cited works according to the standard used by the US National Library of Health and the NIH, where the author originally researched the studies. The publisher is solely responsible for the revision.

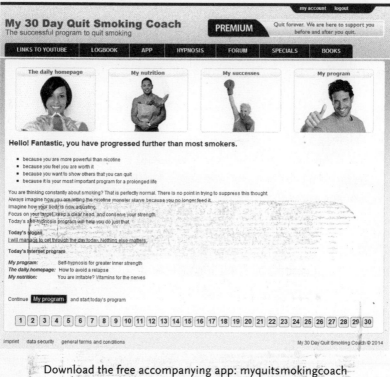

My 30 Day Quit Smoking Coach
The successful program to quit smoking

PREMIUM

Quit forever. We are here to support you before and after you quit.

my account   logout

| LINKS TO YOUTUBE | LOGBOOK | APP | HYPNOSIS | FORUM | SPECIALS | BOOKS |

The daily homepage   My nutrition   My successes   My program

Hello! Fantastic, you have progressed further than most smokers.

- because you are more powerful than nicotine
- because you feel you are worth it
- because you want to show others that you can quit
- because it is your most important program for a prolonged life

You are thinking constantly about smoking? That is perfectly normal. There is no point in trying to suppress this thought.
Always imagine how you are letting the nicotine monster starve because you no longer feed it.
Imagine how your body is now adjusting.
Focus on your target, keep a clear head, and conserve your strength.
Today's self-hypnosis program will help you do just that.

Today's slogan
I will manage to get through the day today. Nothing else matters.

Today's internet program

My program:	Self-hypnosis for greater inner strength
The daily homepage:	How to avoid a relapse
My nutrition:	You are irritable? Vitamins for the nerves

Continue My program and start today's program

1 2 3 4 5 6 7 8 9 10 11 12 13 14 15 16 17 18 19 20 21 22 23 24 25 26 27 28 29 30

imprint   data security   general terms and conditions

My 30 Day Quit Smoking Coach © 2014

Download the free accompanying app: myquitsmokingcoach
Visit the online internet program: www.my30dayquitsmokingcoach.com

About the Author

ANDREAS JOPP is a medical journalist and health coach. He has published 7 internationally bestselling books, which have been translated into 15 languages. Mr. Jopp is also a former smoker and since quitting himself has coached smokers for the last ten years. *I Know You Like to Smoke, But You Can Quit—Now* has been translated into 10 languages and has helped countless smokers worldwide to quit cigarettes for good. For more information visit him at Jopp-online.com or facebook.com/AndreasJopp/en

ACKNOWLEDGMENTS

I would like to thank Colin McCullough for his translation of the book, app, and internet program. This project would not have been possible without his support and friendship. I would like to thank Oliver Fuxen for the creation of the whole manuscript; Iris Bass for her great editing; Jan Lueg and Sebastian Schneider for their tireless Java Programming of "My 30 day quit smoking coach."